INTEGRATIVE CANCER CARE

The Power of Being Informed

by

Dr. Adam McLeod, ND, BSc (Hons)

Author of Dreamhealer Books and DVDs

Additional copies can be purchased at:
www.yaletownnaturopathic.com
or
www.dreamhealer.com

Published in 2015 by Dreamhealer Inc.
Canadian Cataloging in Publication Data
ISBN 978-0-9869037-1-7
UPC# 748252092694

Dr. Adam McLeod, 2015
Integrative Cancer Care - The Power of Being Informed
Printed and bound in Canada.
First printing July 2015

Acknowledgements

Thank you to my amazing family for all of their support over these years. Without their help none of this would have been possible. I am deeply committed to learning everything possible about cancer so that my patients have the most effective treatment plan possible.

This book is dedicated to everyone fighting cancer.

Also by Dr. Adam McLeod

<u>Books</u>

DreamHealer- A True Story of Miracle Healing

DreamHealer- A Guide to Healing and Self-Empowerment

The Path of the DreamHealer

Intention Heals - A Guide and Workbook

<u>DVDs</u>

Visualizations for Self-Empowerment

Heal Yourself

All of the above may be ordered through
www.dreamhealer.com
Books are also available at your local bookstore.

Table of Contents

About the Author

Dr. Adam McLeod is a Naturopathic physician with a special focus on integrative oncology. He graduated with a first class honours degree in molecular biology and biochemistry. He then went on to graduate from Boucher Institute of Naturopathic Medicine as a Naturopathic doctor. Adam is the author of five international best-selling books detailing the discovery of his ability to facilitate a person's natural healing potential. He has spoken at conferences around the world about the science behind the healing power of focused intentions. Dr. McLeod incorporates his molecular biology background to develop targeted integrative cancer protocols for his patients. He firmly believes that a successful evidence-based treatment plan addresses all aspects of the patient's health: physically, emotionally and spiritually. Currently he practices at Yaletown Naturopathic Clinic in Vancouver, British Columbia.

http://www.yaletownnaturopathic.com

Introduction

"Every human being is the author of their own health or disease."
- Buddha

Now is the time that you, as an informed cancer patient, can become involved in your own treatment plan. It is possible to safely and effectively combine natural treatments with conventional therapies to optimize outcomes. This book is an essential guide for all cancer patients who choose to be actively involved in their own health care decisions. By learning about natural evidence-based therapies you can become an empowered patient and make informed decisions about your health.

My journey to integrative oncology was set in motion from a young age. When I was 14 years old I started having undeniable experiences with energy and this led me down the path to becoming an energy healer. I published my first book entitled, *Dreamhealer* at the age of 16 and the response was overwhelming. Over the next 12 years I spoke to thousands of people at conferences around the world to share my experiences with energy healing. It has been a great honour and privilege to have met so many wonderful people at these conferences. As time progressed I began to focus more on how patients can directly influence their own health using their own intentions. Although I was getting excellent results as a healer, I knew that energy healing was not the answer to everything.

I quickly became drawn to molecular biology in an effort to understand the connection between energy and biology. I eventually went on to graduate with a degree in molecular biology and biochemistry which gave me a great knowledge base; but it failed to connect this information to a clinical setting. This amazing journey naturally drew me to Naturopathic medical school where I learned how to apply this knowledge to benefit patients. What is so incredible about Naturopathic physicians is how large our tool box is. We can write conventional prescriptions or order lab tests if it is indicated. We can also use natural remedies to give the body the support that it needs to heal itself. As a Naturopathic doctor I have been able to combine my intuition and energy healing with all the amazing tools that Naturopathic medicine has to offer.

Introduction

Every day I see cancer patients who are looking for natural ways to treat cancer. The truth is that there are many different therapies that are effective at treating cancer. The key to success is using the right combination of therapies at the right time. Everything in this book is for information purposes only. You must consult with a health care professional to determine if these therapies are appropriate for you. By health care professional, I do not mean the person working at the health food store or your friend who consults Dr. Google. Although they may have some helpful information, they do not have the training to understand how all of this works in the complicated clinical context of cancer. Although Medical doctors are an integral part of your health care team, they simply do not have the required training in nutrition or supplements.

These critical areas are not yet part of the standard medical school curriculum. Consequently, a Medical doctor's default answer is often "avoid all supplements," even though this is not what the scientific literature says on the subject. Thus if you have a cancer diagnosis, it's important to consult a licensed Naturopathic doctor whose training provides expertise in nutrition and supplements, and who will then include this knowledge in the practice of integrative oncology.

This book is meant as a guide to focus on evidence-based natural medicine and how it can be used to fight cancer. My goal is to help you sift through the massive amount of information regarding therapies to show you which ones are actually supported by evidence. This book will cover everything from chemotherapy to energy medicine and it will give you a general overview of when to use these different therapies. These cancer therapies are very effective when used appropriately under the guidance of an experienced Naturopathic doctor. The therapies described in this book are only a small fraction of available integrative cancer therapies. This book does not cover every therapy available nor would that necessarily be helpful. By that I mean that a patient should not assume that simply adding additional approaches is always helpful. The body is only capable of absorbing so many things and a simple targeted plan is usually best.

Integrative cancer care begins on the first day of diagnosis and it should continue for the rest of your life. Do not wait until all conventional options are exhausted before seeking integrative care. It is absolutely essential that these integrative protocols are used from the beginning. Your treatment plan does not end when you are cancer free. You must continue to use every tool at your disposal to prevent cancer from recurring. This involves changes in your lifestyle and utilizing targeted supplementation that can be easily implemented for an extended period of time. The goal is not to use a therapy for a few weeks and then never do anything beyond that point. The goal is to establish a simple treatment plan that you can maintain for the rest of your life.

Introduction

Many patients tend to have a dogmatic view when it comes to integrative oncology. Some will immediately have a visceral response against any chemotherapy, radiation or surgery. Others will reject any natural therapy because they are not aware it is evidence-based or because of concern about potential interactions with conventional therapies. The best treatment plan lies in between these two extreme views. The most effective strategy is taking an integrative approach which means that conventional medical treatments are used in conjunction with the appropriate natural therapies. Not only do these natural therapies have important anti-cancer functions, they can also help to support patients through aggressive conventional therapies by substantially reducing side effects.

Ultimately the patient needs to choose a treatment plan that resonates with them. I truly believe that whatever treatment the patient chooses is the right one, even if it is a treatment plan that I disagree with. It is not my job to force the patient to start a treatment plan that they disagree with. It is my job to present the patient with information; then he or she can make an informed decision about their own health and choose the treatment plan that best resonates with them.

An experienced Naturopathic doctor can act as an advocate for your health and ensure that you do not fall through the cracks of the conventional health care system. For example, I have personally witnessed the situation on several different occasions where patients have had an investigative procedure performed.

The results clearly stated that a concerning lesion required additional tests. This concern was not properly communicated to these patients and they got the impression that everything was fine. No one followed up with them, and months later, it turned out that the lesion was indeed cancerous and it had since metastasized.

These cancerous cells could have been easily cured if the patient had been treated in a timely manner. However, since the cancer had spread during unnecessary delays this dramatically reduced the chances of a cure. If these patients had been under the care of a Naturopathic physician at the time, they would have been encouraged to follow up on this report which clearly stated that further investigation was needed. It is the Naturopathic physician's job to make sure that the patient is getting the care they need and that they do not get lost in the system.

Because of my deep commitment to evidence-based treatment, I have taken great care to make sure the approaches discussed in this book are very strongly supported by scientific evidence. For those in doubt, feel free to check out the numerous references throughout this book. All of these references are peer reviewed from well established medical or scientific journals. Integrative oncology is a rapidly evolving field and I am sure that future editions of this book will change as our knowledge evolves.

I am constantly striving to keep up with the research to give my patients the most effective treatment plans possible. In order to effectively battle cancer, we need to constantly modify and adapt our treatments to optimize the chances of success. At the end of the day, my goal is to have looked thoroughly at every component in each patient's life and to suggest the modifications which will give their cells the tools necessary to fight cancer.

Chapter 1

What is Cancer?

"It is more important to know what sort of person has a disease than to know what sort of disease a person has."
- Hippocrates

Some of my first experiences with cancer were as a young teenager experimenting with energy medicine. Cancer patients from around the world were seeking my help and I was surrounded by this disease on a regular basis. There were many cases where I would work with a patient and I literally had no understanding about the biology of the disease. All I knew was that it was clear that the energy was not moving smoothly in one particular area of the body. I would regularly find myself drawn to an area on someone's body and I could not explain why. When I made changes in how the energy was flowing, often the patient started feeling better. This simplistic understanding made it easier to work with cancer from a young age. Even though I knew little about biology, I felt that I had a deep energetic understanding of cancer.

As I started to learn more about biology, my understanding of cancer and energy began to rapidly evolve. Energy is an integral part of the healing process and I have had many experiences where simple changes to energy have resulted in a profound biological response. We like to think of cells as being mechanical units that mindlessly perform tasks, but every cell in your body (including cancer cells) are unique energetic beings. In order to effectively fight cancer, we must learn more about the biology and energy of the disease.

When dealing with a serious illness such as cancer, it is very important to understand the basic biology of the disease. It is essential that you understand what is happening in your own body. You do not have to be a world-class expert on the disease, but you should understand enough so that you can make more informed decisions about your health. This chapter will give you a basic understanding about the development of cancer and the mechanisms that are used to fight these abnormal cells.

Your cells are constantly being damaged. This is unavoidable as oxygen itself will react with essential components in your cells. Our cells have been evolving for billions of years to adapt to these different stressors, and they are remarkably efficient at repairing damage to DNA. Every cell in your body devotes a significant amount of resources to repairing this constant DNA damage. Normally this is relatively insignificant but sometimes this DNA damage starts to accumulate beyond repair. When parts of the cell get damaged that are involved in DNA repair, the cell suddenly becomes less efficient at repairing itself. As a consequence, this DNA damage continues to accumulate and the cell becomes progressively abnormal.

Fortunately our bodies, being multicellular organisms, have developed a powerful molecular pathway to deal with these abnormal cells. When a cell becomes too abnormal, it will recognize that there is a problem and will undergo a process called programmed cell death. In other words, the cell recognizes that it is becoming abnormal, so it shuts down and recycles itself for the benefit of the entire organism.

A cancerous cell is a cell that has gone rogue. It is a cell that is no longer responding to the signals being sent from the body. The cell is trying to go through the process of programmed cell death, but the pathway is defective. Often the goal of chemotherapy and radiation is to damage those cancerous cells just a little bit more so that the signal for programmed cell death gets through.

Every type of cell in your body has the potential to become cancerous. As you can imagine, there are hundreds of potential pathways that can lead to the development of cancer in the body. Each type of cancer will have unique characteristics, which changes the approach to treatment as the therapeutic targets will change. There are a number of hallmark characteristics of cancer which allow it to evade the immune system and invade tissues within the body. It is helpful to break down these features of cancer so that you can better understand your adversary.

The first hallmark characteristic of cancer is that it will grow independently of growth signals. Healthy cells will respond to specific cellular signals and they will not grow or proliferate unless they receive signals to do so. Cancer cells are independent of growth-promoting signals, meaning that they will continue to grow even in the absence of growth signals. Cancer cells are also unresponsive to growth-inhibiting signals. Healthy cells will grow until they physically contact other cells. When the cell is adjacent to another cell, this physical contact will send a powerful signal which will stop the cell from growing. This is how the cells detect if the environment is too crowded. These growth-inhibitory signals allow normal cells to work together as functioning organs. Cancer cells do not respond to this growth inhibition, and they will continue to grow even if they are physically contacting adjacent cells.

This lack of growth inhibition makes it possible for the cancer to invade adjacent tissues. The cells are able to invade deep into the tissues and eventually spread to distant locations throughout the body. Cancer cells are capable of doing this because they do not stop growing when they are adjacent to other cells.

When a normal cell begins to accumulate mutations and becomes more abnormal, a process called apoptosis is triggered. In other words (as described above), when a cell begins to transform into a cancerous cell it recognizes that it is becoming abnormal and it destroys itself. The cell will kill itself because it recognizes that it has the potential to be detrimental to the whole organism. Cancerous cells, on the other hand, are resistant to apoptosis. They have mutated in such a way that this metabolic pathway is defective, and the cell is unable to destroy itself. Cancer cells are actually trying to kill themselves, but for whatever reason the signal for cell death is not being properly recognized.

A normal human cell will only divide a certain number of times before it loses the ability to divide (this is called the "Hayflick Limit"). This is a brilliant mechanism that makes it less likely for cells to become abnormal. Every time a cell divides, there is a chance that an error in the cell division process could result in an abnormal cell. Cancer cells do not adhere to this cell division limit and they are often referred to as "immortal," meaning that they will continue to divide and not adhere to the Hayflick Limit. A good example of this is with HeLa cells, which are commonly used in cancer research. These ovarian cancer cells were cultured from a woman named Henrietta Lacks in 1951, and they continue to grow today because they are immortal. They are still used today in cancer research centres around the world.

Cancer cells grow faster than normal cells, and as a result they need a constant supply of nutrients. They will often secrete chemical signals that trick the body into growing blood vessels into the tumour. This constant blood supply allows the cancer cells to continue their rapid growth. In an effort to sustain this rapid growth, the cancerous cells also fundamentally change their metabolism. They shift their energy production from requiring oxygen (aerobic respiration) to being independent of oxygen (anaerobic respiration). When cells use oxygen to make energy, it is a very efficient mechanism; when they begin to rely on anaerobic respiration, it is incredibly inefficient.

Due to the fact that cancer cells have high metabolic requirements and that they rely on this inefficient energy production, they are wasteful and produce a significant amount of lactic acid. The cancer is essentially burning through all these nutrients inefficiently before normal cells get the opportunity to utilize the nutrients.

One of the biggest challenges in the battle against cancer is that the immune system is not effectively engaging the abnormal cells. Cancer cells have mutated in ways that allow them to avoid detection from the immune system. Once the immune system recognizes the problem, it is very effective at dealing with it. However, often the cancer has mutated to avoid detection by suppressing the immune system. A major focus in current drug development is stimulating the immune system to be more actively engaged in the fight against cancer.

Your immune system is incredibly effective when it recognizes and engages cancerous cells. The goal of any treatment plan is to get the immune system to more effectively recognize these abnormal cells. One technique to stimulate the immune system is to have patients do a series of mental visualizations each day which are described in more detail in chapter 9 (*Intentions and Cancer*). Focused visualizations are a useful tool for sending the message to your cells about where they need to focus their attention. Your cells respond powerfully to the messages that they receive from your mind. This is an innate healing tool that we all possess.

By regularly doing these visualizations, you are sending the message to your cells that this is where they need to pay attention and this can help to increase the activity of your immune system. This is a useful adjunctive cancer therapy that every patient should do on a regular basis. At the end of the day we want to use every tool possible to stimulate the immune system and get it focused on healing. Visualizations and focused intentions are just another tool that can be used to promote the healing process.

Mutation in Cancer Cells

Cancer cells are abnormal on the metabolic and genetic levels and these abnormalities have allowed them to survive in the presence of the immune system. Due to these abnormalities, they are very inefficient at repairing damage to their DNA. This results in a rapid accumulation of genetic mutations. In a normal cell this is undesirable but in a cancer cell this is an essential component to their survival. In fact, cancer cells often sequester iron to help increase the rate of mutations to their DNA. This allows the cancer cells to survive in a wide range of environmental conditions.

A tumour has billions of cells all lumped together, but these cells are not all the same. Of course they share certain characteristics but they have been mutating independently from each other. This is called tumour heterogeneity, which means that there is actually a significant amount of genetic diversity within every tumour. This genetic diversity presents as a huge problem when trying to combat the cancer with chemotherapy.

The cancer may respond well to a specific type of chemotherapy but given the diversity of cells within a tumour it is likely that some of those cells will be resistant to that drug. This is why patients will often see a rapid decrease in tumour mass when they start conventional drug therapies. Many of the cancer cells are initially vulnerable to a specific type of chemotherapy. After several rounds of the chemotherapy the masses often stop shrinking and this is because all the vulnerable cells have been killed. The only cells that remain are the ones that are resistant to the drug. Essentially the chemotherapy was rapidly selecting for cells that are resistant to it. If the drug regimen is not changed then you will often see the cancer come back with a vengeance.

The treatment plan must take into account the fact that these cells are constantly mutating. If you are given one drug, then it is extremely likely that some of the cells within the tumour will mutate to be resistant to that drug. If you analyze the tumour and know that the cells are vulnerable to three or four specific drugs, then your chances of success are much better when they are used simultaneously. The probability of a cell mutating to become resistant to all four drugs at the same time is very low.

Chemotherapy is an effective tool at killing cancer cells when it is used appropriately. The biggest challenge is knowing which drug is best suited for an individual's cancer. Over the years we have learned that certain cancers tend to be more vulnerable to specific chemotherapies. This has resulted in specific protocols being assigned to patients in a "cookie cutter system". For example, if you have Hodgkins lymphoma you are given ABVD[1]. If you have Non-Hodgkins lymphoma you are given CHOP[2]. This model is currently the standard of care with cancer treatment, but it is clear that this is not the most effective way to treat cancer.

It is true that certain cancers tend to be susceptible to certain chemotherapies but these generalizations are not universally correct. There is an incredible degree of variation between cancer cells in different people. Genetic variations are significant even between different cells within one tumour in an individual[3]. In fact, often there is a protocol different than the standard chemotherapy regimen that would be more effective[4]. Unless tests are done, there is no way of knowing which protocol will be the most effective. It is essential to run these tests first and have a clear rationale for the chemotherapy protocol rather than testing it on the patient through trial and error.

There is no question that targeted cancer therapies are the future of oncology. It is important for patients to realize that we already have the ability to do this. Personalized cancer therapy is available, but oncologists rarely encourage it due to the cost. Although these tests are often not covered by insurance, they can be done privately for a few thousand dollars. This is something that patients need to ask for before the surgery. You cannot ask for it to be done afterwards, because the cells will not be adequately preserved. This service is rarely offered to patients and few are even aware that this is an option. You need to specifically ask for the cells to be sent to a lab that runs these special tests.

The cancerous cells will be tested against hundreds of different types of chemotherapies and clear evidence will be obtained about which drugs the cancer is actually susceptible to. This vulnerability of the cancer is determined by an actual test on the cells rather than making generalizations based on the type of cancer. As these tests become more affordable, it will inevitably become the future standard of care because it is so much more effective than the current standard model.

The older chemotherapy protocols use extremely toxic compounds that target any cell which is growing rapidly. In recent years, there have been major advances in drugs that target specific pathways in cancer cells[5]. Before using these targeted drugs effectively it is essential to know which targets the cancer cells are vulnerable to.

Personalized cancer therapy gives patients many additional treatment options. If they do not tolerate the initial chemotherapy regimen well, or if the cancer becomes resistant to the first line therapy, then there is a potential plan B based on molecular evidence. By running this test, it will give your oncologist data that justifies the use of a unique protocol, which may deviate from the current standard of care. The data will give a distinct molecular profile of the cancer that allows a customized treatment plan to be developed for you. If this customized approach is something that you are interested in doing, make sure that you talk to your oncologist. Any Naturopathic doctor who works with oncology on a regular basis will also be familiar with these tests.

Summary:

- Cancer cells are rogue cells which are no longer responding to the signals from the body

- These abnormal cells are inefficient and they use excessive amounts of nutrients from the blood

- There is significant genetic diversity within a tumour as every cell is mutating independently of each other

- The immune system is often not adequately engaging cancerous cells

- Seek integrative care immediately when given the diagnosis of cancer

- Incorporate focused intentions into your treatment plan to send a signal to your immune system about where it needs to focus

- Consider specialized tests on cell samples (if applicable)

References:

1. Bonadonna, Gianni, et al. "Combination chemotherapy of Hodgkin's disease with adriamycin, bleomycin, vinblastine, and imidazole carboxamide versus MOPP." *Cancer* 36.1 (1975): 252-259

2. Fisher, Richard I., et al. "Comparison of a standard regimen (CHOP) with three intensive chemotherapy regimens for advanced non-Hodgkin's lymphoma." *New England Journal of Medicine* 328.14 (1993): 1002-1006.

3. Ross, Douglas T., et al. "Systematic variation in gene expression patterns in human cancer cell lines." *Nature genetics* 24.3 (2000): 227-235.

4. Strickland, Stephen A., et al. "Correlation of the microculture-kinetic drug-induced apoptosis assay with patient outcomes in initial treatment of adult acute myelocytic leukemia." *Leukemia & lymphoma* 54.3 (2013): 528-534.

5. McDermott, Ultan, and Jeff Settleman. "Personalized cancer therapy with selective kinase inhibitors: an emerging paradigm in medical oncology." *Journal of Clinical Oncology* 27.33 (2009): 5650-5659.

What is Cancer?

Chapter 2

Diet and Cancer

**"Let food be your medicine and
your medicine be your food."**
- Hippocrates

When I first started practicing as a Naturopathic doctor, I knew that cancer would be my focus. I began this career thinking that there must be an ideal diet that exists for cancer patients. My view on this has evolved rapidly as I accumulated experience working with cancer. I will always remember one of my first patients, a young man who had recently been diagnosed with cancer. He was otherwise healthy and he strictly adhered to a healthy diet. He could not understand why the cancer continued to progress at such a rapid rate despite his consistently healthy diet and lifestyle. At first I could not understand why the disease was progressing so rapidly when this patient was apparently doing all the right things.

At the same time, I had another patient who was eating all the wrong things. This patient would not change his diet and there was no way to change his mind. He was incredibly stubborn and I found this frustrating as I was constantly looking for ways to help him even though he was unwilling to change his habits. But as time went on, it became apparent that his cancer was not progressing. The disease had stabilized despite this patient apparently doing all the wrong things. This was the complete opposite of my other patient who was deteriorating despite doing everything right.

After sitting down and reflecting on these two cases, it became clear to me what the critical difference was between these patients. The patient eating all the wrong foods had no fear of the foods that he was eating or of the cancer. He was perfectly content to eat these foods even at the risk of worsening the disease. He was simply not concerned about the effects that food would have. The patient eating all the right things was very concerned about the foods that he was putting into his body. He thought that he must be doing something wrong as this would be the only explanation for the progression of the disease. He obsessed over every item that he consumed. It was not the food that was the problem. It was the fear that was the problem. The worst thing that you can eat is fear.

Of course these are two extreme examples and I am not downplaying the significance of diet and cancer. I believe that diet is an important component of a comprehensive cancer treatment plan. That being said, the most essential thing to eliminate from your diet is fear. Do not fear the foods you eat. You must whole-heartedly embrace the foods you eat as nutrients for your heart and soul.

When given a serious diagnosis such as cancer, patients often immediately resort to the internet for information and they quickly become overwhelmed. It becomes a real challenge for patients when everyone they talk to suggests a different therapy and they hear conflicting opinions on a daily basis. When developing a comprehensive treatment plan a good place to start is your diet. It is helpful to take a close look at the foods that you are putting into your body. By modifying your diet appropriately this can make a major difference both in how you feel and in the effectiveness of therapies used. There are countless different diets and supplements that are promoted for their anti-cancer effect. It is impossible to choose among them by yourself. You must have professional guidance to develop a diet and supplement plan to fight cancer safely and effectively.

I have great respect for Medical oncologists and the work that they do. We all need to make more of an effort to work collaboratively because we all have effective tools to offer patients. Every day I see cancer patients who were told by their oncologist to avoid Naturopathic medicine because those therapies can interfere with chemotherapy or even promote the growth of cancer. Many doctors refuse to collaborate in any way with Naturopathic physicians because Medical oncologists have literally no training in these natural approaches. They simply tell patients to avoid them all with the implication that they are dangerous. This fear-mongering has to stop.

Of course you have to be careful about what you put into your body when you are fighting something serious like cancer. Naturopathic doctors who regularly work with oncology are aware of these dangerous interactions. We have extensive training in these therapies and we will not give the patient something that has a dangerous interaction with chemotherapy or radiation. When Naturopathic therapies are used appropriately, patients do much better. These treatments are also very strongly supported by scientific evidence.

The most commonly used therapies by Naturopathic physicians have literally hundreds of peer reviewed studies demonstrating their effectiveness and safety when used in conjunction with conventional therapies. The examples cited of negative interactions between natural therapies and conventional medications were often not prescribed by Naturopathic doctors. Unfortunately in some states and provinces, Naturopathic medicine is not regulated; as a consequence anyone in these unregulated areas can call themselves a "naturopath" or a "Doctor of Natural Medicine". A "Doctor of Natural Medicine" is merely a trademark and is not a designation recognized under the Health Professions Act. This confuses both the public and some members of the mainstream medical community.

A Naturopathic doctor is someone who, after receiving an undergraduate degree, has attended another four years of medical school. Having studied both pharmacology and natural supplements, Naturopathic doctors are very familiar with these drug interactions. Believe me, when ANY negative interaction with natural therapies is discovered, the medical community is very quick to point it out. As a result, we are acutely aware of such interactions and we only use therapies that have a demonstrable safety record.

Naturopathic medicine has a wide range of tools that can be used in conjunction with conventional medicine to effectively treat cancer. Many people have the faulty assumption that Naturopathic treatments are not "evidence-based" because otherwise their oncologist would have recommended them. The truth is that Naturopathic therapies used by competent certified Naturopathic doctors are extremely well documented by scientific studies, and the mainstream scientific community does not dispute their effectiveness. The bottom line is that cancer patients do better when they have an integrative health care team and Naturopathic doctors are an integral part of this team. When dealing with a complex condition such as cancer, it is important to thoroughly review the entire health history of the patient, not just the diagnosis of cancer.

It is essential that as physicians we actually take the time to listen to what the patient is saying. This allows us to develop a custom treatment plan for each individual which addresses the unique circumstances of that patient. Naturopathic doctors are experts at taking the time to listen to the patient and developing a treatment plan for each unique patient.

Chemotherapy and radiation are effective therapies, but often it is a race between the death of the cancer cells and the death of healthy cells. Making sure the healthy cells are supplied with adequate nutrients allows patients to endure these conventional therapies with fewer side effects. Often patients who are adequately supported with the appropriate nutrition and supplements will be able to tolerate additional rounds of chemotherapy and radiation. Ultimately if healthy cells are more likely to survive, this helps stack the odds against cancer cells surviving.

Patients are often reluctant to take any supplements during chemotherapy and radiation because of potential interactions. This is a legitimate concern because there are many negative interactions if the wrong supplement is used. Naturopathic doctors who regularly work with cancer are well aware of these interactions. When the appropriate supplements are used there are profound benefits to cancer patients. These supplements are well supported by scientific literature and they have been consistently demonstrated to be safe when used in the right context. This is why the blanket statement of "avoid all supplements" is simply incorrect.

It is absolutely essential that you have professional guidance from an experienced Naturopathic doctor when you are choosing supplements. The mainstream medical community is slowly becoming more open to collaborating with Naturopathic doctors because the evidence for the benefits of an integrative approach to cancer care can no longer be ignored. There are many dietary and supplemental changes that have consistently demonstrated a synergy with conventional treatments.

With all this information available about diet and supplements, it is easy to focus entirely on physical components of the disease, and by doing so, the emotional components of healing become neglected. There is no question that there is often a strong emotional component to cancer and this must be addressed for optimal healing to take place. Patients will often be able to directly connect the formation of their cancer with a stressful event in their life. There are biological reasons why emotional stress can trigger the formation of cancer.

The link between cancer and stress is well-known. Many people are not aware of how significant this connection is. Even Medical doctors often disregard this connection despite the body of evidence. A good physician will not only address the physical components of health, they will also take the time to address the emotional and spiritual components that simply cannot be ignored in patients with cancer.

This chapter will briefly summarize some of the most commonly recommended dietary changes used in integrative oncology. To fully implement these diets, you will need the guidance of an experienced health care professional. If you know someone with cancer, make sure you let them know about the potential benefits of seeing a Naturopathic physician. There are so many amazing tools that Naturopathic medicine has to offer, and the public needs to be aware that these therapies exist and that they are effective!

Diet during Chemotherapy and Radiation

The vast majority of my patients tell me that their doctor bluntly told them that it doesn't matter what they eat during their chemotherapy or radiation treatments. Some of these physicians are so locked into this belief that they give zero dietary advice because they are convinced that diet will not make a difference.

Diet and Cancer

As a molecular biologist, this disregard for diet made no sense to me. During these aggressive therapies such as chemotherapy and radiation, every cell in the body is under an enormous amount of stress. The metabolic demands on your cells are obviously increased so that they can survive in the presence of these toxins. If the metabolic demands are increased, then the cells clearly need nutrients to supply this demand. There is a big difference between the nutrient content of a Twinkie and an apple. Logic dictates that this difference in nutrients should make an even bigger difference when your cells are bathed in chemotherapy and radiation in an effort to kill cancer.

Could all of these oncologists be wrong? They are highly educated and if they feel so passionately about the role of diet (or lack thereof) in cancer, then surely there must be a scientific reason for this. I decided to look at peer-reviewed articles that study how diets affect patients during chemotherapy and radiation. It turns out that this attitude from oncologists is not based on logic or scientific fact. The evidence is clear; diet makes a big difference when patients are on chemotherapy and radiation. Doctors who claim to be practicing evidence-based medicine need to reconsider the practice of telling patients that diet makes no difference, because this is not what the evidence shows.

Many studies have been done on humans and rats, which clearly show positive effects from diet during chemotherapy. One simple study clearly demonstrated that when given a diet that is rich in nutrients, rats are able to tolerate significantly higher doses of chemotherapy and radiation[1,2]. This is consistent with the ultimate goal of keeping your cells strong so that the patient can better tolerate chemotherapy. If your cells are stressed, then they will need more nutrients to deal with that stress. By eating foods that are nutrient dense, it allows the cells to adapt to the stress of chemotherapy and radiation more effectively.

There are several diets which have been shown to be clearly synergistic with chemotherapy, including caloric restriction. Caloric restriction is a method where the patient maintains their nutrient status while decreasing the number of calories that they are ingesting. A recent article in the journal *The Oncologist* breaks down the different mechanisms showing how caloric restriction can enhance the effects of chemotherapy and radiation[3]. The conclusion of their research was:

> Caloric restriction by fasting is likely an effective method to potentiate the cytotoxicity of chemotherapy and radiation therapy because of the overlapping induction of molecular profiles, and it may also provide a beneficial means of improving the overall health and metabolic

profiles of patients. At this time, clinical trials evaluating caloric restriction as a complementary therapy in the treatment of cancer are warranted. (Champ et al. 101)

Another diet which is effective with certain cancers is the ketogenic diet. The positive effects from this diet are not debated in the scientific community. Pilot trials have also been completed on the ketogenic diet and how it affects the quality of life in advanced cancer patients. The results clearly show that specific diets such as this can improve quality of life in these patients[4]. These are just a few brief examples of how different diets can impact your health during chemotherapy and radiation.

Fasting before Chemotherapy

There has been a major movement lately for cancer patients to fast before and after an infusion of chemotherapy. When first hearing this, it is counter-intuitive. It sounds like a horrible idea to encourage a patient to fast when their body is already stressed with chemotherapy but fasting before chemotherapy has been used safely in several clinical trials[7,10]. It turns out that there is a significant amount of scientific data to support this therapy when the patient is properly supervised. This is an interesting shift in thinking, because the conventional approach in the past has been to encourage patients to get as many nutrients into their body as possible.

There are a number of metabolic reasons why fasting may increase the effectiveness of chemotherapy while reducing the side effects[8,9]. It turns out that fasting triggers normal cells to enter into a protective mode. They rapidly become more efficient and this triggers a reduction in glucose and Insulin-like growth factor 1 (IGF-1) levels by more than 50%[9]. This rapid metabolic shift would be very difficult to achieve even with a potent mixture of drugs. Cancer cells are unable to shift into this protective mode thus making them more vulnerable to the chemotherapy than normal cells[11]. This is referred to as differential protection, and it has the potential to transform conventional cancer care.

The preferred length of fasting before chemotherapy varies significantly in the trials done so far. The most commonly recommended fasting period is 48 hours before chemotherapy and this continues until 24 hours after the chemotherapy infusion. During this fasting period, ideally the patient should have only water. They should be as close to complete fasting as possible. Although it is clearly uncomfortable not eating for a total of 72 hours, research indicates that this is a worthwhile sacrifice. The discomfort from hunger will actually decrease the severity of the side effects from the chemotherapy. This starvation state is triggering a powerful metabolic shift in your cells which protects healthy cells while making the cancer cells more vulnerable to the chemotherapy.

As fasting before chemotherapy is further researched, it is likely that other mechanisms will be discovered that explain this differential protection. Even without a fully defined biochemical mechanism for this protection, it is clear that fasting does make a substantial difference. Do not implement a fasting protocol before chemotherapy without the supervision of a qualified health professional. Fasting before chemotherapy is completely contraindicated with several common diseases such as diabetes. It is essential that you are monitored during this process because fasting is not safe for everyone.

Diet alone is not a cure for cancer but when used properly it can help patients maintain their nutrient status during chemotherapy and radiation. I know that oncologists sincerely want the best for their patients and I have great respect for the work that they do. However, when they are asked about diet it is probably better that they say, "I don't know" rather than "don't waste your time with diets because it won't make a difference." Unfortunately, oncologists do not get sufficient training in nutrition and its role in cancer therapy. Their lack of training in nutrition is apparent when you consider their position on the subject despite the evidence showing that it can be an effective tool[6].

The bottom line is that diet does make a difference. This is what the evidence shows. There is no question that a healthy balanced diet will make it easier for patients to tolerate chemotherapy and radiation. Even though many of these patients have low energy levels during chemotherapy, research indicates they are willing and able to adhere to specific diets during chemotherapy[5]. Anyone who eats a low quality diet will have lower energy and consequently a poorer quality of life (recall the movie *Supersize Me*). This is common sense and this concept obviously applies to those who are undergoing conventional cancer treatments. It is not uncommon in my practice for patients to be going through chemotherapy and radiation with minimal side effects because they are nutritionally supported during this process. If you eat a high quality diet under the supervision of a Naturopathic doctor, then your cells will be better nourished to deal with the stresses of cancer and the aggressive treatments.

The Myth of the Alkaline Diet

I often see cancer patients who are drinking alkaline water and focusing a significant amount of their time and energy on alkaline foods. Is this an effective diet in the fight against cancer? The short answer is no and any observed positive effects have nothing to do with the foods being alkaline. Let me explain why this is so.

In the early 20th century, it was observed that cancer cells could not grow in alkaline environments. There are a number of metabolic reasons why this is so, and this theory is effective in a petri dish. The problem is that this theory simply does not apply to our bodies. The pH is a measure of how acidic or basic (alkaline) a liquid is. You cannot change the pH of your blood enough to influence cancer. To understand why, you need to look at the biochemistry of the blood.

Our blood is buffered, which means that it is absolutely full of molecules that ensure there are no variations in the pH of the blood. The body spends a substantial amount of energy keeping the pH of the blood within a very narrow range. Every single protein in your entire body is designed to work at a specific pH. If there is any deviation from this optimal pH, then the proteins will cease to function properly. In other words, if you were able to make your blood significantly more basic it would quickly result in kidney failure, respiratory failure and ultimately death.

Our cells have been adapting to a narrow pH range for millions of years and there are many metabolic reasons for this. When you drink alkaline water and eat alkaline foods, it does not make your blood alkaline. When you increase consumption of alkaline food and water it will make your urine and saliva more basic. The reason that these fluids become more basic is because your body is working hard to excrete these basic molecules so that your blood pH remains the same.

In other words, if your urine or saliva is more basic this does not mean that your blood pH has changed to any significant degree. Any positive studies relating to the alkaline diet have nothing to do with the foods being alkaline. When you look at the list of "alkaline foods," it consists mostly of fresh fruit, vegetables, nuts and legumes with small amounts of meat. These are all healthy foods that are rich in nutrients. It is this high nutrient content that is giving patients health benefits. The high nutrient content is completely unrelated to the alkaline nature of these foods.

When designing an ideal diet plan for cancer patients, the first goal is to make sure they are getting adequate nutrients because the cells will have increased metabolic demands while fighting cancer. The second goal is making sure that they are avoiding foods that are rich in sugar. Often this diet will consist of fresh fruits, vegetables, nuts and legumes. No one disputes that these foods are helpful when combating cancer but it is clear that this positive effect is not due to them being alkaline.

The Ketogenic Diet

The ketogenic diet is commonly used to treat epilepsy, and it also appears to have applications in an integrative cancer setting as well. The concept behind this diet is that by changing the composition of the foods you eat it will fundamentally change the energy metabolism in your nervous system. This diet consists of consuming high fats while avoiding carbohydrates. The ketogenic diet can be a challenge to maintain, but in specific cases it is certainly worth the effort.

This high fat and low carbohydrate diet forces the body to burn fats for energy rather than sugars. Normally the brain uses glucose (sugar) as its primary source of energy, but if there is a shortage of sugar, the liver then converts fats into ketone bodies. These ketones pass into the brain and replace glucose as the primary source of energy. High levels of ketones in the blood are strongly correlated with a decrease in the frequency of epileptic seizures[11].

Healthy cells within the nervous system are able to easily shift their metabolism to become dependent on ketone bodies. Cancerous cells within the nervous system have high energetic requirements and they struggle to shift to this new energy source. As a result, cancers that are of nervous tissue origin are vulnerable to the ketogenic diet. The ketogenic diet slows down the rate of growth of brain tumours because the cancerous cells do not have an abundant and usable energy source under these conditions[13,14,15].

In my experience, the ketogenic diet works synergistically with dichloroacetic acid (DCA) in patients with brain tumours. The evidence for the use of the ketogenic diet with brain cancers is overwhelming. There is also evidence to suggest that this diet can be helpful with other forms of cancer[16]. However, the impact of the ketogenic diet on other forms of cancer is certainly not as dramatic as its effect on brain tumours.

This diet is difficult to maintain for long periods of time; it takes discipline to do it properly. I always recommend the ketogenic diet to patients with brain cancers; however, I do not regularly recommend it to patients with other forms of cancer. Although there is some evidence to suggest that it can still be helpful, it is often very stressful for patients to adhere to this strict diet plan. In advanced metastatic cases, it can be helpful to begin the ketogenic diet because it slows down the rate of tumour growth by changing the energy source for the cancer. In localized cancers that do not originate from the nervous system, the effect of the ketogenic diet is minimal. This diet is not a cure for cancer but it can certainly help to slow the growth and it can be used safely in conjunction with other medical treatments.

In order for this diet to have the desired effect, you need to strictly adhere to the diet plan. The goal is to starve the cancer cells of their primary energy source. Every time you consume sugar, the cancer cells will immediately use this to produce energy. There are a number of good online resources that can help you transition to an effective ketogenic diet.

I regularly update helpful links on the clinic website (*www.yaletownnaturopathic.com*) that will direct you to accurate and current resources.

It will require strong willpower and self-control to adhere to this diet plan effectively. Often when making such a dramatic dietary change, the key to success is slowly transitioning to the new diet. In this circumstance, however, it is best to make the transition as rapidly as possible. Resources like the trusted links on my website can help with that transition. It is important to consult a Naturopathic doctor because this diet is not for everyone and it takes clinical judgment to determine if this is the best option for you.

Red Meat and Cancer

Many people have heard that you should avoid red meat when battling cancer. Several different large studies have consistently demonstrated a correlation between red meat consumption and an increased risk of developing cancer[17,18,19]. The reason for this connection is that red meat is rich with a molecule called heme. When heated this can form molecules known as heterocyclic amines. These heterocyclic amines are suspected carcinogens that are formed in meat when it is cooked at a high temperature for long durations. It is thought that the metabolism of this molecule leads to a highly cytotoxic factor in the colonic lumen, which increases the generation of free radicals. Although studies consistently blame the heme molecule for the carcinogenic effect of red meat, it is clear that this negative effect cannot be fully attributed to this one molecule[18]. In addition to heme, red meat has high levels of IGF-1, free iron and omega-6 fatty acids. These molecules may also contribute to the carcinogenic effect of red meat.

It turns out that some people are more susceptible to the negative effects of red meat than others. People with a mutation in genes called NAT1 or NAT2 are much more likely to develop colon cancer if they consume red meat[17]. These enzymes activate the carcinogenic heterocyclic amines that are commonly found in red meat. When these molecules are activated they are more likely to damage the DNA in the colon epithelium.

The connection between red meat and colon cancer is clear and the mechanism is relatively well defined. The carcinogenic effects of red meat are not localized exclusively to the colon. Regular consumption of red meat also significantly increases the risk of developing breast cancer[21] especially in premenopausal women. Consumption of red meat is strongly correlated with the development of estrogen positive and progesterone positive breast cancer[20]. It is likely that this increased risk of breast cancer could also be attributed to the highly carcinogenic heterocyclic amines.

Diet and Cancer

There are many people who have made the argument that corn-fed red meat is associated with an increased cancer risk but that grass-fed meat is safe. The research clearly demonstrates that grass-fed has a higher nutritional content and is rich in many molecules that are associated with a decreased cancer risk[23]. There is no debating that grass-fed is healthier for you than corn-fed. Nevertheless, I am not convinced that grass-fed red meat is safe for cancer patients. Just because one is healthier than the other does not mean that it is safe for cancer patients. I would be hesitant to include red meat in any cancer diet plan even if it is grass-fed. One exception to this rule is in patients who are very anemic and present with consistently low levels of iron.

The bottom line is that if you are fighting cancer or eating healthy to prevent the recurrence of cancer, then you should make an effort to avoid red meat. Not only is consumption of red meat associated with cancer but it is clear that people who avoid red meat and consume other protein sources have a lower risk of developing cancer[22]. There are many different delicious and healthy sources of protein that can replace red meat. This simple dietary shift is something that every cancer patient (especially breast and colon cancer patients) should seriously consider.

Glycemic Levels and Cancer Recurrence

I tell virtually every cancer patient that they should avoid sugar as much as possible. Some doctors insist that sugar has no effect on cancer. This is simply not what the scientific literature states. If you are trying to fight cancer or prevent the recurrence of cancer, then you should make an effort to reduce your sugar intake.

Study after study has demonstrated a direct connection between sugar intake and cancer risk[24,25,26,27,28]. There are a wide range of cancers which are associated with increased sugar intake. Cancer cells often have significantly more insulin receptors than normal cells. In other words, they respond very rapidly to insulin and they will always be more effective at grabbing sugar from the blood stream and utilizing it as an energy source. Cancer cells will always grab the sugar before normal cells due to this fundamental shift in their metabolism.

The sugar acts as a direct source of energy for the cancer cells. These abnormal cells are often dependent on a constant supply of sugar, which is pushed through anaerobic glycolysis to provide them with energy. Essentially the sugar acts as fuel which directly stimulates the growth of cancerous cells. The fundamental challenge is that normal cells also require sugar and it is simply not possible to eliminate sugar completely.

It turns out that although sugar acts as fuel to cancer cells, the mechanism for the enhanced tumour growth from sugar is different than you would expect. There is a big difference in the metabolism of a food rich in simple sugars compared to a food that contains complex carbohydrates. When you eat a food rich in simple sugars such as candy, the body rapidly absorbs the sugar. This causes a rapid and significant elevation of the sugar concentration in your blood. In response to this sugar spike, the pancreas secretes insulin, which circulates through the entire body in an effort to bring the sugar levels back to normal.

Insulin interacts with the receptors on the surface of both normal and cancerous cells. Upon interacting with the cells, it helps them to pull sugar in from the blood until the blood sugar level drops back to a normal level. Remember that cancer cells have more insulin receptors, so they will always take advantage of this insulin spike more effectively than normal cells. It is this spike in insulin and insulin-like growth factors that stimulate the growth of cancerous cells[25]. In other words, it is not the sugar content that is stimulating growth; it is the response to sudden increases in sugar levels.

Complex carbohydrates (commonly found in many foods such as lentils, beans and quinoa) are metabolized differently in the body. They do not cause a sudden spike in blood sugar levels. The sugar in complex carbohydrates is slowly released as the food passes through the gastrointestinal tract. As the sugar is being slowly released, it is also being metabolized by cells within the body at a similar rate. As a result, it is not necessary for the pancreas to secrete as much insulin because there is no spike in blood sugar that needs to be controlled.

Despite the overwhelming evidence, some skeptical health care professionals insist that avoiding sugar makes no difference because everything we consume has sugar in it. Although it is true that virtually everything we eat contains some sugar, this simple logic is completely incorrect and demonstrates a lack of understanding of the mechanism. The sugar is not directly stimulating the growth of cancer, but there is no question that our body's response to sugar does stimulate cancer.

Sugar, Inflammation and Recurrence

There are several key metabolic changes that occur in the body when exposed to simple sugars such as in candy. High levels of sugar in the blood seem to inhibit the function of the immune system and stimulate inflammation[28,29]. This inflammation is not localized; it is a true systemic inflammatory response. There are countless studies which strongly suggest that chronic inflammation is a significant factor in the development and in the progression of cancer. This inflammatory response makes it easier for cancer cells to evade detection by the immune system and it enhances the rate of spread. Any effective cancer treatment plan must address systemic inflammation and make a significant effort to control it in a balanced way.

Obviously when fighting cancer, it is critical to use every tool at your disposal to keep the immune system strong so that it can focus on the task at hand. Hyperglycemia (high levels of sugar in the blood) inhibits the function of the immune system on a number of different levels. It is important to recognize that this immune suppressing effect is not something that would be readily detected from any blood work. The number of white blood cells and neutrophils in the blood will remain the same, however, these cells will not be working as effectively. The immune cells will not attack cancer cells as effectively when they are exposed to high levels of sugar.

It is logical that if sugar inhibits the immune system and stimulates inflammation, then you would expect high levels of sugar to be associated with an increased cancer risk. The correlation between high glycemic diets and cancer risk is well established. It is essential that patients looking to prevent recurrence of cancer adhere to a low glycemic diet.

There was a recent study conducted on women with a history of breast cancer. In this study researchers looked for a connection between fasting blood glucose levels and risk of cancer recurrence. There was a strong correlation between high fasting blood glucose levels and cancer recurrence[30]. In other words, the women who consistently had high levels of sugar in their blood had a higher risk of developing cancer. This is really not surprising given what we know about the relationship between sugar and cancer.

The connection between sugar and cancer is both logical and well supported by data. What can be done to decrease the levels of sugar in the blood? The safest approach is making modifications to your diet so that you are not putting large amounts of sugar into your body in the first place. Start reading labels and become familiar with the foods that you are putting into your body. If it looks sugary and tastes sugary, then it is probably sugary and it is best to avoid it. The first step is obvious; avoid putting simple sugars into your body. Beyond dietary modifications there are a number of different pharmaceutical options, the most common being metformin, which is associated with a decreased cancer risk (although the mechanism for this anti-cancer effect may not be related to sugar).

Another helpful dietary change is increasing your fibre intake. When you consume fibre, it essentially slows the release of sugar into the blood stream. This results in less insulin being secreted and consequently less stimulation of any residual cancer cells. The data on fibre consumption and cancer prevention is mixed but generally positive. In one large study on fibre intake and breast cancer recurrence (known as the HEAL cohort), it was determined that fibre decreased risk of recurrence, but the improvement was not considered statistically significant[30]. Another study concluded that higher levels of fibre consumption provided significant benefit to overall survival, but this benefit was not necessarily related to cancer[31].

Many patients immediately focus on avoiding gluten when they get the diagnosis of cancer. It is important to mention that avoiding gluten is not usually a critical component of a diet designed to fight cancer. Generally speaking you want to avoid foods that will stimulate inflammation in the body and in some people consumption of gluten certainly triggers a systemic inflammatory response. Patients who are sensitive to gluten should certainly make an effort to avoid it. In those who are not particularly sensitive to gluten, going gluten-free is not the number one priority. We have to focus on getting the essential nutrients into the cells so that they can more effectively fight the cancer.

It is also worth pointing out that many of the gluten-free foods are high in sugar. In many of the better tasting gluten -free products, there are significant amounts of sugar added. In the context of cancer, this added sugar will cause more problems than any benefit that would be gained from the absence of gluten. If avoiding gluten makes you feel healthier and more vital then by all means avoid it. It is critical to recognize that just because it is gluten-free does not mean that it is healthy. You need to make a conscious effort to avoid sugar and read the labels of the foods that you are putting into your body.

The sugar content of fruits is generally not a concern. In my experience, most patients could benefit from having more fruits in their diet. Any negative impact from the sugar in fruits is far outweighed by the positive effects of the nutrients and the natural antioxidants. There are some fruits which are exceptionally rich in sugar. These sugar rich fruits such as mangos, kiwis, bananas and dried fruits should be consumed in moderation. It can be helpful to look at the glycemic load (not the glycemic index) of your favourite fruits and modify your diet accordingly to reduce your intake of sugar. It is not necessary to strictly avoid these sugar rich fruits but by eating them in moderation you can substantially reduce your overall sugar consumption.

The bottom line is that it is not hard to connect the dots. Consuming high levels of sugar has a number of effects on the body. Sugar promotes inflammation, weakens the immune system and stimulates the growth of cancerous cells. If patients consume a low glycemic diet, then they are less likely to develop cancer and any cancer cells that are present will not grow as quickly. Fibre helps to further enhance a low glycemic diet by reducing your body's response to sugar. At the end of the day the goal is to develop a diet plan that you can maintain for the rest of your life. There is no benefit adhering to a strict diet for only a short period of time. When it comes to cancer prevention, it is best to develop a simple and sustainable long-term treatment plan that you can easily maintain.

Natural Antioxidants during Chemotherapy

I was very surprised to hear a patient tell me that their doctor told them to specifically avoid blueberries. This was the only dietary recommendation they were given. When I asked why the doctor prescribed such a bizarre dietary change, the patient replied that the antioxidants from blueberries can interfere with the chemotherapy and radiation. Although I was happy to hear that this doctor was offering dietary advice, unfortunately this advice is not accurate.

There is no evidence to suggest that antioxidants from natural sources are dangerous during chemotherapy or radiation. In fact, virtually all of the literature clearly states that it is beneficial to get antioxidants from natural sources. By consuming antioxidant rich foods, patients have fewer side effects during conventional cancer treatments. Many studies have also clearly demonstrated that these foods do not interfere with the effectiveness of these therapies[34,35,36,37,38,39].

It is interesting to note that of all the foods in the world, this doctor picked only one item: blueberries. I am not sure of the rationale for this recommendation because there are countless foods that have antioxidant properties. Although blueberries are commonly associated with being antioxidants, they are not very potent when compared to many other common foods.

The antioxidant capacity of a food is measured by a lab test which determines the ability of that food to neutralize free radicals. This is commonly known as the Oxygen Radical Absorbance Capacity (ORAC) and a quick Google search will clearly demonstrate that blueberries do not even make the top 50 for antioxidant capacity. These values are based on biological samples *in vitro* and it is not clear how significant these values are in the human body. What is clear, however, is that ORAC values are a measure of the antioxidant capacity of these foods.

Depending on the source that you use, blueberries have a ORAC value of approximately 6,500 which is not particularly high when compared to cinnamon with an ORAC value of 265,000. This means that cinnamon is approximately 40 times more powerful as an antioxidant than blueberries. Of course one could argue that you do not eat as much cinnamon as blueberries, which is indeed true. However, there are other foods consumed in comparable amounts to blueberries which have a significantly higher antioxidant capacity. Unsweetened cocoa powder has an ORAC value of 81,000 and baking chocolate has an ORAC value of 50,000. If you are having a food rich in chocolate, then chances are you are consuming more antioxidants than if you are having blueberries[33,40].

I am not suggesting that chocolate should be a primary source of antioxidants. I would certainly prefer that my patients get their antioxidants from blueberries rather than chocolate. There are many bioflavonoids in blueberries that are helpful in the context of cancer. Excessive consumption of chocolate will clearly result in undesirable spikes in blood sugar. The point is that it is silly to single out one food as an antioxidant concern. The reality is that if you really want to cut antioxidants out of your diet it would involve much more than the elimination of blueberries. The advice of avoiding blueberries is confusing and it is simply not an evidence-based dietary plan.

Natural sources of antioxidants are very helpful in the context of cancer and there is no debate about this in the scientific community. The debate is around synthetic supplementation with high doses of antioxidants during chemotherapy and radiation. Natural sources are well established as beneficial in these cases, as they protect healthy cells without interfering with the effects of conventional therapies[37].

Blueberries are a great source of nutrients and they provide a balanced antioxidant support that is synergistic with chemotherapy and radiation. What is particularly interesting is that wild blueberries are much more effective at neutralizing free radicals than cultivated blueberries. Depending on which measurements you use, in some cases the wild blueberries have almost double the antioxidant capacity. So make sure you eat your blueberries and give your cells the nutrients they need!

Summary:

- Seek professional guidance to develop an effective diet plan that you can maintain for a long period of time

- Stick to a low glycemic diet and avoid simple sugars

- Sugar from fruit is generally not a concern although fruits with a high glycemic load should be consumed with moderation

- Consume adequate amounts of antioxidant rich foods and fibre

- Avoid red meat especially in cases of colon and breast cancer

- Fast 48 hours before chemotherapy and 24 hours after (if indicated)

- Strictly adhere to the ketogenic diet if it is a tumour of neurological origin

- It is not necessary to focus on the pH of the food and water that you consume

References:

1. Bounous, G., et al. "Dietary protection during radiation therapy." Strahlentherapie 149.5 (1975): 476-483

2. Branda, Richard F., et al. "Diet modulates the toxicity of cancer chemotherapy in rats. *Journal of Laboratory and Clinical Medicine* 140.5 (2002): 358-368. Champ, Colin E., et al. "Nutrient restriction and radiation therapy for cancer treatment: when less is more." *The Oncologist* 18.1 (2013): 97-103.

3. Champ, Colin E., et al. "Nutrient restriction and radiation therapy for cancer treatment: when less is more." *The Oncologist* 18.1 (2013): 97-103.

4. Schmidt, Melanie, et al. "Effects of a ketogenic diet on the quality of life in 16 patients with advanced cancer: A pilot trial." *Nutr Metab (Lond)* 8.1 (2011): 54.

5. von Gruenigen, Vivian E., et al. "Feasibility of a lifestyle intervention for ovarian cancer patients receiving adjuvant chemotherapy." *Gynecologic oncology* 122.2 (2011): 328-333.

6. Rock, Cheryl L., et al. „Nutrition and physical activity guidelines for cancer survivors." CA: a cancer journal for clinicians 62.4 (2012): 242-274. Safdie, Fernando M., et al. "Fasting and cancer treatment in humans: A case series report." *Aging (Albany NY)* 1.12 (2009): 988.

7. Safdie, Fernando M., et al. "Fasting and cancer treatment in humans: A case series report." *Aging* (Albany NY) 1.12 (2009): 988.

8. Raffaghello, Lizzia, et al. "Fasting and differential chemotherapy protection in patients." *Cell Cycle* 9.22 (2010): 4474-6.

9. Lee, C., and V. D. Longo. "Fasting vs dietary restriction in cellular protection and cancer treatment: from model organisms to patients." *Oncogene* 30.30 (2011): 3305-3316.

10. de Groot, S., et al. "Abstract P4-16-12: CARE: A pilot study of the effects of short-term fasting on tolerance to (neo) adjuvant chemotherapy in breast cancer patients." *Cancer Research* 73.24 Supplement (2013): P4-16.

11. Laviano, Alessandro, and Filippo Rossi Fanelli. "Toxicity in chemotherapy—when less is more." *New England Journal of Medicine* 366.24 (2012): 2319-2320.

12. Freeman, John M., Eric H. Kossoff, and Adam L. Hartman. "The ketogenic diet: one decade later." *Pediatrics* 119.3 (2007): 535-543.

13. Zhou, Weihua, et al. "The calorically restricted ketogenic diet, an effective alternative therapy for malignant brain cancer." *Nutr Metab (Lond)* 4.5 (2007): 5.

14. Nebeling, Linda C., et al. "Effects of a ketogenic diet on tumor metabolism and nutritional status in pediatric oncology patients: two case reports." *Journal of the American College of Nutrition* 14.2 (1995): 202-208.

15. Seyfried, Thomas N., and Purna Mukherjee. "Targeting energy metabolism in brain cancer: review and hypothesis." *Nutrition & metabolism* 2.1 (2005): 30.

16. Schmidt, Melanie, et al. "Effects of a ketogenic diet on the quality of life in 16 patients with advanced cancer: A pilot trial." *Nutr Metab (Lond)* 8.1 (2011): 54.

17. Chen, Jia, et al. "A prospective study of N-acetyltransferase genotype, red meat intake, and risk of colorectal cancer." *Cancer research* 58.15 (1998): 3307-3311.

18. Sesink, Aloys LA, et al. "Red Meat and Colon Cancer The Cytotoxic and Hyperproliferative Effects of Dietary Heme." *Cancer research* 59.22 (1999): 5704-5709.

19. Lewin, Michelle H., et al. "Red meat enhances the colonic formation of the DNA adduct O6-carboxymethyl guanine: implications for colorectal cancer risk." *Cancer research* 66.3 (2006): 1859-1865.

20. Cho, Eunyoung, et al. "Red meat intake and risk of breast cancer among premenopausal women." *Archives of internal medicine* 166.20 (2006): 2253-2259.

21. Zheng, Wei, et al. "Well-done meat intake and the risk of breast cancer." *Journal of the National Cancer Institute* 90.22 (1998): 1724-1729.

22. Pan, An, et al. "Red meat consumption and mortality: results from 2 prospective cohort studies." *Archives of internal medicine* 172.7 (2012): 555-563.

23. Daley, Cynthia A., et al. "A review of fatty acid profiles and antioxidant content in grass-fed and grain-fed beef." *Nutrition journal* 9.1 (2010): 10.

24. Augustin, L. S. A., et al. "Dietary glycemic index and glycemic load, and breast cancer risk: a case-control study." *Annals of Oncology* 12.11 (2001): 1533-1538.

25. Franceschi, S., et al. "Dietary glycemic load and colorectal cancer risk." *Annals of Oncology* 12.2 (2001): 173-178.

26. Michaud, Dominique S., et al. "Dietary sugar, glycemic load, and pancreatic cancer risk in a prospective study." *Journal of the National Cancer Institute* 94.17 (2002): 1293-1300.

27. Gnagnarella, Patrizia, et al. "Glycemic index, glycemic load, and cancer risk: a meta-analysis." *The American journal of clinical nutrition* 87.6 (2008): 1793-1801.

28. Qi, Lu, and Frank B. Hu. "Dietary glycemic load, whole grains, and systemic inflammation in diabetes: the epidemiological evidence." *Current opinion in lipidology* 18.1 (2007): 3-8.

29. Turina, Matthias, Donald E. Fry, and Hiram C. Polk Jr. "Acute hyperglycemia and the innate immune system: clinical, cellular, and molecular aspects." *Critical care medicine* 33.7 (2005): 1624-1633.

30. Belle, Fabiën N., et al. "Dietary fiber, carbohydrates, glycemic index, and glycemic load in relation to breast cancer prognosis in the HEAL cohort." *Cancer Epidemiology Biomarkers & Prevention* 20.5 (2011): 890-899.

31. Kroenke, Candyce H., et al. "Dietary patterns and survival after breast cancer diagnosis." *Journal of clinical oncology* 23.36 (2005): 9295-9303.

32. Contiero, Paolo, et al. "Fasting blood glucose and long-term prognosis of non-metastatic breast cancer: a cohort study." *Breast cancer research and treatment* 138.3 (2013): 951-959.

33. Haytowitz, David B., and Seema Bhagwat. "USDA database for the oxygen radical absorbance capacity (ORAC) of selected foods, Release 2." *US Department of Agriculture* (2010).

34. Moss, Ralph W. "Should patients undergoing chemotherapy and radiotherapy be prescribed antioxidants?." *Integrative cancer therapies* 5.1 (2006): 63-82.

35. Simone, Charles B., et al. "Antioxidants and other nutrients do not interfere with chemotherapy or radiation therapy and can increase kill and increase survival, part 1." *Alternative therapies in health and medicine* 13.1 (2007): 22.

36. Drisko, Jeanne A., Julia Chapman, and Verda J. Hunter. "The use of antioxidant therapies during chemotherapy." *Gynecologic oncology* 88.3 (2003): 434-439.

37. Moss, Ralph W. "Do antioxidants interfere with radiation therapy for cancer?." *Integrative cancer therapies* 6.3 (2007): 281-292.

38. Conklin, Kenneth A. "Cancer chemotherapy and antioxidants." *The Journal of nutrition* 134.11 (2004): 3201S-3204S.

39. Block, Keith I., et al. "Impact of antioxidant supplementation on chemotherapeutic toxicity: a systematic review of the evidence from randomized controlled trials." *International Journal of Cancer* 123.6 (2008): 1227-1239.

40. Vertuani, Silvia, et al. "Evaluation of Antiradical Activity of Different Cocoa and Chocolate Products: Relation with Lipid and Protein Composition." *Journal of medicinal food* 17.4 (2014): 512-516.

Chapter 3

Intravenous Therapies and Cancer

"You can be a victim of cancer or a survivor of cancer. It's a mindset."
- Dave Pelzer

Early in my career as a Naturopathic doctor, I had a patient who was given only a few months to live and he presented at my office with a diminished vitality. He was dementias, confused and unable to communicate in a coherent manner. The patient was primarily interested in intravenous therapies to treat his cancer. I started the patient on IV Vitamin C and after a few short weeks he started to look more vital. Suddenly he was able to carry on conversations and we got to see his personality. He was a friendly old man who lit up the clinic with his humour and his positive energy. All the staff always looked forward to seeing him whenever his name was on the schedule.

As the therapies continued he was progressively looking better and better. His dementia had significantly improved and he had a strong sense of vitality. This continued several months beyond the "expiry date" that he was given by his oncologist. Although he was feeling great, he wanted to get another CT scan to help assess the effectiveness of the treatments. The results of the scan were not positive and I was responsible for sharing this new information with him for the first time. When I explained that the mass had advanced, I could see in his eyes that he lost the will to fight at that very moment. The fact that he was feeling great and living beyond expectations did not matter to him. He interpreted these results as a sign that the therapy was not working.

After this visit he went to see his oncologist who looked at the results and then looked back at the patient and said, "I don't care what these results say; you are looking great, so whatever you are doing, just keep doing it." It was good to hear these words of encouragement from the oncologist, but it was not enough to change the patient's mindset. He had decided after seeing these results that he did not want to fight anymore and he died soon after this. The entire clinic was deeply saddened by the news of his passing. We had all come to know this patient very well and we all miss his uplifting humour.

A couple of weeks after his passing, his son came to the clinic to let us know how grateful the family was for our help. The patient was commuting around the city and shopping on his own until two weeks before his passing. There is no doubt that these therapies helped the patient to feel better and live longer even in this advanced stage of cancer. This touching case taught me two things. It clearly demonstrated the power of intravenous therapies in a case where there was little hope and few options available.

This experience also reinforced the importance of having the will to fight and how a negative result can crush that will. I will always remember that moment when I looked into his eyes as I gave him the bad news. I knew in that moment that he was not going to fight anymore. Although scans are helpful and they provide critical information, you cannot focus entirely on the measurements and the numbers. An important measurement, which we cannot quantify effectively is how you feel. If you are feeling well and living longer, then that is a huge success, regardless of what any scan or test says.

Intravenous therapies can be a very effective tool because the human body is only capable of absorbing so many things. Sometimes it is best to bypass this absorption issue and infuse compounds directly into the blood. There are many different natural therapies which can be used intravenously. These therapies can range from a basic nutrient cocktail that supports a malnourished patient, to intravenous DCA that is used in combination with a select few chemotherapies. An experienced health care professional will be able to develop a unique protocol that addresses the specific concerns with each case. In this chapter, I will discuss a number of different intravenous (IV) therapies which are commonly used in an integrative cancer setting. There are many other therapies which can be administered intravenously, but the ones discussed here are the most common and they are well supported by scientific evidence.

High Dose IV Vitamin C

High dose intravenous Vitamin C as an anti-cancer therapy has gained a lot of attention in the media lately. There is no doubt that when used appropriately this can be an effective integrative cancer therapy[1]. As the evidence mounts, mainstream medicine is slowly beginning to embrace high dose IV Vitamin C.

When taken orally at low doses Vitamin C is an effective antioxidant and it has many positive health benefits in the context of general health. Oncologists will frequently tell their patients to fear antioxidants because they will neutralize the effects of the chemotherapy. Their rationale is that chemotherapy works by adding oxidative stress to cancer cells and antioxidants will neutralize this effect. On an intuitive level this makes sense, but the majority of the scientific evidence indicates that when used appropriately, antioxidants protect healthy cells without interfering with the effects of the chemotherapy[2,3].

The important point here is that Vitamin C is not an antioxidant when given at high doses intravenously[4]. Strangely enough, at high doses, IV Vitamin C switches roles and acts as a potent oxidative molecule, which is the complete opposite of its antioxidant role at lower doses. Studies show that at high doses IV Vitamin C is very toxic to cancer cells[6]. In this cellular context it is a potent oxidative molecule that works synergistically with most conventional therapies.

Patients who undergo this therapy tend to experience fewer side effects from the chemotherapy[7,8]. IV Vitamin C can vastly improve quality of life by increasing appetite, raising platelet counts, easing fatigue and reducing pain. Studies consistently show that at these high doses, IV Vitamin C is toxic to cancer cells while protecting healthy cells from the effects of chemotherapy. The evidence indicates that IV Vitamin C is effective when used in conjunction with chemotherapy rather than as a stand-alone therapy.

There are several different situations where high dose IV Vitamin C is not safe. Although it is safe to use with most chemotherapies, it is not safe to use with Velcade (Bortezomib)[5]. There are a number of studies that show a negative interaction between this particular drug and Vitamin C. When injecting Vitamin C there is a significant amount of sodium that is in the infusion and this can be a heavy burden on the kidneys. This stress to the kidneys is only a concern in patients that have significantly compromised kidney function.

Even with patients who have normal kidney function, it is important to stay hydrated during the IV Vitamin C infusion. There is a substantial amount of salt being put directly into the veins and your cells will be thirsty even if you do not feel a sense of thirst.

There is also a rare genetic condition known as G6PD and in these patients it is not safe to administer high doses of Vitamin C. It is always best to check for this mutation even though it is quite rare. It is necessary to have an experienced health care professional to assess your health history and ensure that you do not have any contraindications to this therapy.

One important factor that more doctors need to become aware of is that it is not necessary to add B-vitamins to the IV Vitamin C. This was added in the past because the logic was that these patients are very depleted and in need of additional B-vitamins. This is indeed true. Many of these patients are in need of B-vitamins because of the extreme stress on the cells. However, there is evidence that suggests the addition of B-vitamins is actually counter-productive and it reduces the potency of the Vitamin C. In other words, if the fluid in the bag is yellow then it was not mixed correctly. The fluid in the bag should be transparent. If you are in need of B-vitamins, then it should be administered separately rather than mixed with the Vitamin C.

It is also important to point out that when IV Vitamin C is administered to patients, it will affect blood sugar readings. The ascorbic acid is similar to glucose on the molecular level, so diabetic patients will often test their blood sugar after an infusion and get a false high reading. Some patients see this high glucose reading and immediately give themselves insulin to bring down blood sugar levels. The problem is that this is a false reading. Their blood sugar levels are not high; they just appear to be high based on the test. Consequently, when the patient administers insulin under these conditions, their blood sugar can drop to dangerously low levels. It is essential that diabetic patients be made aware of this interaction and that they factor this in before they administer insulin.

All patients, including patients who are not diabetic, should stay hydrated and eat snacks during an IV Vitamin C infusion. This ensures that the blood sugar remains balanced and it reduces the risk of dehydration. There is a lot of salt in a bag of IV Vitamin C. Attached to every molecule of ascorbic acid is two sodium molecules, so you have to stay hydrated. I regularly run IV Vitamin C on my patients at the clinic and it is an effective cancer therapy when used appropriately. On a regular basis, I see patients improve significantly when they use this therapy as part of a comprehensive integrative cancer protocol.

Before starting IV Vitamin C patients need to review their finances to see if this treatment plan is realistic. Generally speaking IV Vitamin C must be looked at as a long-term therapy. The vast majority of the positive clinical trials on IV Vitamin C are when it is administered several times per week over the course of several years. It is not an effective therapy if patients just get the IV a few times. At approximately $150 per IV, the costs begin to add up very quickly. It is important to recognize that IV Vitamin C is not the only therapy available and it is not necessarily the most effective treatment in every case. There are many other more cost effective therapies which can be used if Vitamin C is too expensive.

Much of the debate about IV Vitamin C revolves around the cost-to-benefit ratio of the therapy. It is clear that it makes a positive difference, but some oncologists argue that the observed benefit is not worth the high cost of using this therapy long-term. A good Naturopathic physician should help you develop a plan that is both effective and fits within your budget. Although integrative cancer care can often be pricey, a more expensive treatment plan is not necessarily more effective. The most effective treatment plan often consists of just a few targeted supplements that are specific to a patient's unique health concerns.

Intravenous Artesunate and Iron Deficiency

Everyone has seen someone with cancer who looks pale and depleted of energy. This is often due to anemia, which means that there are fewer red blood cells to transport oxygen to tissues in the body. There are a number of potential causes for this and one of the most common reasons is low iron. When a doctor looks at blood work that clearly says "low ferritin", there is often an immediate response to supplement the patient with iron. We should not be so quick to prescribe iron to every cancer patient that is showing signs of anemia.

The interactions between iron and cancer are very complex and altered iron metabolism is considered a key metabolic "hallmark of cancer"[14]. It is clear that iron has roles in all aspects of cancer development, including the tumour microenvironment and metastasis. As evidenced by the expression pattern of iron genes in malignant tumours, altered iron metabolism is not simply associated with cancer but also is indicative of a patient's chances of survival[15].

Our bodies have evolved to tightly partition and limit the amount of available iron. The iron deficiency anemia that is observed in cancer patients may actually be the body's response to the presence of cancer. By limiting the availability of iron in circulation, there is less available for the cancer to utilize. If the patient is given iron, then you are essentially fighting against the body's effort to lower the iron levels.

There are a number of different studies that clearly show a strong connection between low iron levels and decreased cancer risk. It is well documented that people who regularly donate blood have lower rates of developing cancer[16]. This is likely connected to decreased iron levels following donation of blood. A popular natural cancer therapy called curcumin acts as a potent natural chelator of iron[18]. It is thought that some of the observed anti-cancer properties might be due to the fact that it powerfully sequesters iron away from cancer cells[19].

Recent research indicates that tumours create their own iron-rich microenvironment to evade constraints that are imposed by limited systemic iron availability. Cancer cells will sequester iron and it is possible that this allows the cancer cells to mutate more quickly. Iron reacts with oxygen to produce free radicals that damage DNA. Normally this is not desirable; however, this allows cancer cells to adapt more quickly to different conditions when the DNA is being constantly damaged on a low level. This consistent damage from excess iron is thought to increase the mutation rate of the DNA within the cancer cells. The regulation of iron in the tumour microenvironment represents a new paradigm in iron biology[17].

Of course there are some situations where iron must be prescribed, but it should not be done unnecessarily. Many effective cancer therapies work by actually decreasing the level of iron in the blood. If the red blood cells are reduced in number and smaller than normal (low MCV) then you most likely have iron deficiency anemia. It is important to also check the level of ferritin to assess your body's ability to transport iron. There is a potent intravenous therapy called artesunate, which can take advantage of the iron metabolism of cancer.[12]

Artesunate is a drug that was initially designed for combating malaria. However, recently it has shown great promise as a cancer therapy[8,9,10]. It has been used in combination with some chemotherapies to improve outcomes in advanced cancer patients[5]. When fighting cancer, it is important to use every tool at your disposal to weaken the cancer and strengthen your own cells. Artesunate is another weapon in the arsenal of natural remedies that can make a significant difference in the fight against cancer.[13]

The mechanism of action for artesunate in the context of cancer therapy is well defined. Cancer cells have a tendency to absorb iron at high levels and this is thought to accelerate the mutation rate within these cells. In normal cells this reaction is a problem; in cancer cells it allows them to mutate and develop resistance to therapies. Artesunate activates mitochondrial apoptosis by iron catalyzed lysosomal reactive oxygen species production[11]. This means the drug will use the iron within the cancer cells against them.[12]

Preliminary data from Bastyr Integrative Oncology Research Center indicates that IV Vitamin C in conjunction with IV Artesunate makes a substantial difference in advanced cancers. IV Artesunate is often administered right before high dose IV Vitamin C and there is evidence that these therapies work synergistically together. In patients with stage 4 breast cancer, after one year the group that received no IV Vitamin C or IV Artesunate had a 74% survival rate. This compares to the IV Vitamin C and IV Artesunate group which had a 90% survival rate after one year. By year two the results were even more significant as the group that did not receive treatment had a 68% survival rate compared to 90% in the treatment group. It is also important to note that no adverse events were associated with this treatment.

These preliminary results strongly suggest that high dose IV Vitamin C and IV Artesunate improves survival in stage 4 breast cancer patients. Evidence is growing that the use of this therapy is effective for a wide range of cancers. Research has shown that Artesunate can increase quality of life in addition to improving survival rates. Just like any other cancer therapy, it is important that it is used under the supervision of a experienced Naturopathic physician who focuses on oncology.

DCA and Brain Cancers

Several years ago there was a huge buzz in the media about Dichloroacetic Acid (DCA) and its use in cancer[20]. The public was outraged that DCA could be an effective cancer therapy and yet little interest was shown because DCA could not be patented. The drug companies ignored any evidence related to this therapy because without a patent, it was simply not a profitable venture. Fortunately, some private researchers raised enough money to continue studies into this simple yet effective therapy.

DCA was initially used for lactic acidosis, a condition where the blood has high levels of lactic acid. The DCA inhibits an enzyme called pyruvate dehydrogenase kinase, which causes a major shift in metabolism from fermentation to oxidation in the mitochondria[21]. In other words, it forces the mitochondria inside cancer cells to become more active. This is relevant to cancer because the survival of cancer cells depends on the mitochondria being dormant. The mitochondria are capable of triggering cell death in abnormal or damaged cells. Cancer cells are grossly abnormal and they require the mitochondria to be inactive.

The ultimate goal of this therapy is to activate the mitochondria and allow them to trigger cell death in the abnormal cancerous cells. The DCA will certainly help to activate these pathways, but it is essential that patients also exercise. By regularly doing aerobic exercise, you are also stimulating the mitochondria. The excessive energetic demands during exercise trigger the mitochondria to be more active and burn oxygen. DCA when combined with exercise significantly increases the consumption of oxygen by the mitochondria, which is an indication that the mitochondria are being further activated[24].

It is essential for cancer patients (not just patients on DCA) to do aerobic exercise if they are physically able to. The type of exercise does not matter, as long as it is a moderate aerobic exercise that you are able to do on a regular basis. There is an overwhelming body of evidence which clearly shows that cancer patients who regularly exercise simply do much better than those who do not. It is possible that mitochondrial activation could be one of the reasons for this.

Most of the research seems to indicate that DCA is more effective for cancers that are localized in the nervous system[22]. Although it can be used for other types of cancer, it is less indicated for cancers that do not originate from the nervous system. A common side effect from chemotherapy is neuropathy[23] and DCA should be used with caution if there are any signs of neuropathy. The only known drug interaction with DCA is a drug called Lasix which is a diuretic. Overall, DCA is a safe therapy and there are many studies that demonstrate the safety of this therapy.

Based on my experience with DCA, I would only recommend it for cancers which are localized to the nervous system. Brain cancers are dependent on sugar for energy and the DCA seems to be able to exploit this vulnerability. It is particularly effective against brain cancers when DCA is combined with the ketogenic diet (see chapter 2 *Diet and Cancer* for more information on the ketogenic diet). The ketogenic diet is rich in healthy fats while strictly avoiding sugar. It can be challenging to adhere to this diet, but it is well supported in the scientific literature[25,26,27]. Exercise would be a synergistic addition to the combination of a ketogenic diet and DCA, because all of these therapies work together to activate the mitochondria within cancerous cells.

The bottom line is that DCA is an effective therapy when used appropriately. It is not a cure on its own, but DCA can be a major part of a comprehensive treatment plan. It can be administered either orally or intravenously. The oral dose is typically 15-20mg/kg and it is cycled two weeks on followed by one week off. It is extremely important to have the appropriate neurological support during this therapy. DCA is known to cause significant neuropathy and you must be monitored by a physician who is experienced with the use of DCA. Common neurological support includes methylcobalamin (B12), thiamine (B1) and alpha lipoic acid (ALA). It is critical that you consult with a Naturopathic physician who focuses on oncology to know what neurological support is best suited for you.

Intravenous Alpha Lipoic Acid

Alpha lipoic acid (ALA) is an antioxidant that has been used for decades to help with nerve related symptoms of diabetes. It can also be used to treat a long list of conditions including cancer. ALA is a unique antioxidant because due to its molecular structure, it can act as both a fat-soluble and water-soluble antioxidant. This unique property makes ALA a critical component of the antioxidant network. It seems that at high doses, it helps to prevent cell damage and it rapidly regenerates the supply of vitamin E and C.

ALA can either be taken orally or through intravenous therapy. The oral form is well absorbed if it contains the pure R form. The S form of alpha lipoic acid is poorly absorbed and it does not have the same positive effects. It is critical that the oral supplementation consists of the pure R form if you expect to get any positive benefits. When ALA is given intravenously, it is not necessary to differentiate between the R and S form because it is being infused directly into the blood stream. It is important to point out that ALA is very sensitive to light; therefore, the IV bag and the line must be protected from ultraviolet (UV) rays. There are some special bags and lines that are opaque which have UV filters. Most clinics simply wrap the line and the bag in tin foil to preserve the ALA while it is being infused.

The intravenous route allows much higher doses of ALA to be administered, and it is these higher doses that are linked to an anti-cancer effect. It appears that ALA triggers mitochondrial respiration and induces apoptosis in cancerous cells[29]. There are a number of reported cases of long-term disease stabilization with ALA and low dose naltrexone in patients with metastatic pancreatic cancer[30,31]. The exact mechanism for this effect is not known, but in addition to increasing mitochondrial reactive oxygen species, it has also been documented as a p53 activator in cancerous cells[32]. p53 is a tumour suppressor that is commonly inactivated in cancerous cells. By activating this molecule, it triggers programmed cell death in these abnormal cells. At higher doses ALA will compete with B-vitamins (particularly biotin) and this can cause a deficiency if patients are not adequately supported.

Chemotherapy can be hard on the nervous system, and it is not uncommon for patients to develop neuropathy. This can manifest as a sensation of tingling, burning or pain in the hands and feet. Once this neuropathy develops during chemotherapy, it is often irreversible. Recent research indicates that ALA can improve the function and conduction of neurons. This property makes ALA an ideal candidate for nerve support during chemotherapy[28]. In patients who have neuropathy prior to starting chemotherapy, it is important to be proactive with nerve supports. IV ALA can help to support the nerves and reduce the risk of neuropathy developing or progressing during chemotherapy. Due to the fact that ALA is an antioxidant, it is not safe with all chemotherapy protocols. However, there are some chemotherapy regimens where its use is safe and effective.

There are a couple of important details that must be considered when giving patients intravenous alpha lipoic acid. The ALA will potentiate insulin so you must be cautious when administering this to diabetic patients. Although it is not a contraindication to diabetes, you must carefully monitor their blood sugar before you start any infusion. It cannot be mixed with other compounds or it will form precipitates in the bag. It should be administered in a separate bag and the line should be flushed if another solution was given beforehand. For optimal absorption (and safety), it is critical that the ALA be put in a non-ionic solution such as D5W.

Summary:

- IV Vitamin C has a wide range of uses and is synergistic with many types of chemotherapy

- IV Artesunate can be used prior to an infusion of IV Vitamin C and it is particularly useful in cases of sarcomas and breast cancer

- DCA is useful against cancers of neurological origin but this drug can be toxic to the nerves and neurological support is necessary to prevent neuropathy

- IV ALA can be used with pancreatic cancer and it helps to prevent neuropathy induced by chemotherapy

References:

1. Vollbracht, Claudia, et al. "Intravenous vitamin C administration improves quality of life in breast cancer patients during chemo-/radiotherapy and aftercare: results of a retrospective, multicentre, epidemiological cohort study in Germany." *in vivo* 25.6 (2011): 983-990.

2. Suhail, N., et al. "Effect of vitamins C and E on antioxidant status of breast-cancer patients undergoing chemotherapy." *Journal of clinical pharmacy and therapeutics* 37.1 (2012): 22-26.

3. Tabassum, A., R. G. Bristow, and V. Venkateswaran. "Ingestion of selenium and other antioxidants during prostate cancer radiotherapy: a good thing?." *Cancer treatment reviews* 36.3 (2010): 230-234.

4. Carr, Anitra, and Balz Frei. "Does vitamin C act as a pro-oxidant under physiological conditions?." *The FASEB Journal* 13.9 (1999): 1007-1024.

5. Perrone, G., et al. "Ascorbic acid inhibits antitumor activity of bortezomib in vivo." *Leukemia* 23.9 (2009): 1679-1686.

6. Riordan, N. H., et al. "Intravenous ascorbate as a tumor cytotoxic chemotherapeutic agent." *Medical hypotheses* 44.3 (1995): 207-213.

7. Weijl, N. I., et al. "Supplementation with antioxidant micronutrients and chemotherapy-induced toxicity in cancer patients treated with cisplatin-based chemotherapy: a randomised, double-blind, placebo-controlled study." *European Journal of Cancer* 40.11 (2004): 1713-1723.

8. Takemura, Yukitoshi, et al. "High dose of ascorbic acid induces cell death in mesothelioma cells." *Biochemical and biophysical research communications* 394.2 (2010): 249-253.

9. Efferth, Thomas, et al. "The anti-malarial artesunate is also active against cancer." International journal of oncology 18.4 (2001): 767-773.

10. Michaelis, Martin, et al. "Anti-cancer effects of artesunate in a panel of chemoresistant neuroblastoma cell lines." *Biochemical pharmacology* 79.2 (2010): 130-136.

11. Du, Ji-Hui, et al. "Artesunate induces oncosis-like cell death in vitro and has antitumor activity against pancreatic cancer xenografts in vivo." *Cancer chemotherapy and pharmacology* 65.5 (2010): 895-902.

12. Efferth, Thomas, et al. "Enhancement of cytotoxicity of artemisinins toward cancer cells by ferrous iron." *Free Radical Biology and Medicine* 37.7 (2004): 998-1009.

13. Zhang, Z. Y., et al. "[Artesunate combined with vinorelbine plus cisplatin in treatment of advanced non-small cell lung cancer: a randomized controlled trial]." *Zhong xi yi jie he xue bao= Journal of Chinese integrative medicine* 6.2 (2008): 134-138.

14. Hanahan, Douglas, and Robert A. Weinberg. "Hallmarks of cancer: the next generation." *Cell* 144.5 (2011): 646-674.

15. Miller, Lance D., et al. "An iron regulatory gene signature predicts outcome in breast cancer." *Cancer research* 71.21 (2011): 6728-6737.

16. Edgren, Gustaf, et al. "Donation frequency, iron loss, and risk of cancer among blood donors." *Journal of the National Cancer Institute* 100.8 (2008): 572-579.

17. Torti, Suzy V., and Frank M. Torti. "Iron and cancer: more ore to be mined." *Nature Reviews Cancer* 13.5 (2013): 342-355.

18. Jiao, Yan, et al. "Iron chelation in the biological activity of curcumin." *Free Radical Biology and Medicine* 40.7 (2006): 1152-1160.

19. Jiao, Yan, et al. "Curcumin, a cancer chemopreventive and chemotherapeutic agent, is a biologically active iron chelator." Blood 113.2 (2009): 462-469. Coghlan, Andy. "Cheap, safe drug kills most cancers." *New Scientist* 2857 (2007): 13..

20. Coghlan, Andy. "Cheap, safe drug kills most cancers." *New Scientist* 2857 (2007): 13.

21. Stacpoole, Peter W. "The pharmacology of dichloroacetate." *Metabolism* 38.11 (1989): 1124-1144.

22. Michelakis, E. D., et al. "Metabolic modulation of glioblastoma with dichloroacetate." *Science translational medicine* 2.31 (2010): 31ra34-31ra34.

23. Abramowski, M. C. "Chemotherapy-induced neuropathic pain." *J of the Advanced Practitioner in Oncology* 1 (2010): 279-283.

24. Ludvik, Bernhard, et al. "Effects of dichloroacetate on exercise performance in healthy volunteers." *Pflügers Archiv* 423.3-4 (1993): 251-254.

25. Seyfried, Thomas N., et al. "Metabolic therapy: a new paradigm for managing malignant brain cancer." *Cancer letters* 356.2 (2015): 289-300.

26. Chiu, Martina, et al. "Towards a metabolic therapy of cancer?." *Acta bio-medica: Atenei Parmensis* 83.3 (2012): 168-176.

27. Zastre, Jason A., et al. "Linking vitamin B1 with cancer cell metabolism." *Cancer & metabolism* 1.1 (2013): 16.

28. Gedlicka, C., et al. "Effective treatment of oxaliplatin-induced cumulative polyneuropathy with alpha-lipoic acid." *Journal of clinical oncology* 20.15 (2002): 3359-3361.

29. Wenzel, U., A. Nickel, and H. Daniel, "α-lipoic acid induces apoptosis in human colon cancer cells by increasing mitochondrial respiration with a concomitant O2–.-generation." *Apoptosis* 10.2 (2005): 359-368.

30. Berkson, Burton M., Daniel M. Rubin, and Arthur J. Berkson. "The long-term survival of a patient with pancreatic cancer with metastases to the liver after treatment with the intravenous α-lipoic acid/low-dose naltrexone protocol." *Integrative cancer therapies* 5.1 (2006): 83-89.

31. Berkson, Burton M., Daniel M. Rubin, and Arthur J. Berkson. "Revisiting the ALA/N (α-Lipoic Acid/Low-Dose Naltrexone) protocol for people with metastatic and nonmetastatic pancreatic cancer: a report of 3 new cases." *Integrative cancer therapies* 8.4 (2009): 416-422.

32. Simbula, G., et al. "Increased ROS generation and p53 activation in α-lipoic acid-induced apoptosis of hepatoma cells." *Apoptosis* 12.1 (2007): 113-123.

Intravenous Therapies and Cancer

Chapter 4

Chemotherapy Support

"To ensure good health: eat lightly, breathe deeply, live moderately, cultivate cheerfulness, and maintain an interest in life."
- William Londen

It is essential that you whole-heartedly embrace whatever treatment that you choose. When you do this, you will have fewer side effects and the treatment will be more effective. I will always remember the following two cases, because they were so different and they happened at around the same time. One patient was undergoing chemotherapy for pancreatic cancer, and he was given the generally well-tolerated drug gemcitabine. Most patients have minimal side effects with this drug. At the same time, another patient was on a very aggressive chemotherapy protocol for advanced colorectal cancer. He was on some of the most toxic drugs that are associated with horrible side effects.

The patient on the generally well-tolerated drug hated the chemotherapy. He despised the fact that he was on this drug. Even though the side effects from this drug are typically minimal, he was having horrible reactions. Every possible side effect that you could think of was manifesting in this patient. These reactions helped to fuel his hatred for the drug. Not only was he having terrible side effects, the scans indicated that the cancer was not responding nearly as well as expected.

The other patient, who was on the highly toxic chemotherapy had no fear of the drugs and he embraced it as his cure. He went into the treatment with a positive mindset knowing that these toxic drugs would be the answer to his problem. Unbelievably, this patient had virtually no side effects to the drugs. Not only that, the cancer was responding much better than expected, and as of right now, he is cancer free.

I firmly believe that the contrasting attitudes of these patients dramatically influenced their responses to therapy. Although they were taking different drugs for different forms of cancer, in both cases there was such an obvious connection between their attitudes and their clinical response. I have seen many similar cases in my clinic, and when I talk to colleagues they have also observed similar situations. The body's response to one's attitude is not an isolated event. This is a common observation in any clinic that focuses on cancer. The bottom line is that your attitude and mindset going into a treatment make a significant difference. Whatever treatment you are doing, you need to embrace it as your cure.

Many patients are hesitant to begin chemotherapy because they are fearful of the side effects. They are given a long list of potential reactions with no information about how to minimize these side effects. It is true that chemotherapy has side effects, but cancer has side effects too. The good news is that there are many different natural therapies that can act synergistically with these drugs while reducing side effects. It is reassuring for the patient to know that they are doing something to support their health in addition to the chemotherapy. It is extremely important that you have a licensed Naturopathic physician determine if your supplements are indicated or safe for your type of chemotherapy. Every therapeutic approach that is described in this section has potential contraindications if it is not used properly. A Naturopathic doctor will be able to help you develop a plan that is safe and effective for your particular chemotherapy regimen.

I had the privilege of attending the 4th annual Oncology Association of Naturopathic Physicians (ONCANP) conference where Naturopathic doctors from around the world gathered to discuss the latest research and advances in integrative oncology. It is exciting to see how rapidly the field is advancing and much of the information presented can be applied in a clinical setting to anyone battling cancer.

I was interested to learn at the conference that several cancer clinics in the United States have Naturopathic doctors working at hospitals in collaboration with Medical oncologists. The results from this collaboration are nothing short of incredible. When the data is compared to the national standards, it is clear that the patients are living longer with an enhanced quality of life in this integrative cancer setting. One stunning example was with stage 3 lung adenocarcinoma patients where the overall survival was 36 months compared to the national average of around 12 months. Study after study showed that patients were responding more effectively to the chemotherapy and that they were having fewer side effects. I find it extremely frustrating that this integrative model is not universally applied, given the abundance of evidence.

There needs to be a major change in the medical system to embrace this integrative model because the bottom line is that it works. The problem at this point in time is that many Medical oncologists refuse to work at all with Naturopathic doctors. Instead, they tell their patients to avoid all natural supplements because they fear that it will interfere with the conventional treatments. This is simply not true. Moreover, it is easy to find evidence supporting these integrative therapies.

Patients are not stupid. When they are given a serious diagnosis, they turn to the internet in search of answers even if their oncologist says that they are wasting their time. The problem is that patients do not have the medical knowledge to recognize which supplements are appropriate for them and which ones are contraindicated. By telling patients to avoid all supplements and avoid all Naturopathic doctors, this pushes patients to do their own research and they take supplements without informing their oncologist. The reality is that they need professional guidance from a Naturopathic doctor to choose the right supplements and the Naturopathic doctor should then inform the oncologist about the treatment plan that the patient is on. This creates a better healing environment for the patient, and it ensures that everyone is on the same page about the treatment plan.

In the past I have had doctors scare patients about the most benign prescriptions or supplements. Patients have been told that omega-3's will accelerate tumour growth because it is an "antioxidant" or that EGCG "protects cancer cells" in patients not even on chemotherapy. These statements are simply untrue and a quick literature search would reveal dozens of references regarding the safety and effectiveness of these supplements.

I have also had a number of patients who were told to discontinue a prescription of metformin or Celebrex only when the MD found out that a Naturopathic doctor prescribed it. In these cases the patients were responding well to the chemotherapy and they were taking these medications during this entire time period. The pharmacist who filled the prescription didn't have a problem with it and I am sure that had a MD prescribed the exact same thing the oncologist would have never recommended that the patient discontinue it.

Patients should not be put in a position where they are being forced to make decisions based on one health care practitioner creating fear and suspicion about another. This is highly inappropriate. Having said that, I also feel that Naturopathic doctors need to make more of an effort to reach out to Medical doctors. We all need to make more of an effort to act collaboratively for the benefit of the patient.

When I say that we need to move to an integrative model, it should be clear by now that I am not suggesting that patients should avoid chemotherapy. Integrative cancer care means that we use evidence-based treatment plans to work synergistically with conventional medicine. Most of my cancer patients are undergoing chemotherapy or radiation because ultimately patients do best when they are adequately supported through these conventional therapies.

What many Medical oncologists do not realize is that often Naturopathic doctors are encouraging patients to do the same treatment plan that the oncologist recommended. Sometimes an oncologist can unwittingly scare away the patient from conventional therapies simply based on how they describe the treatment. As Naturopathic physicians, we make an effort to educate the patient and give them the support that they need through these conventional therapies. When patients have support they are more likely to follow through with chemotherapy and they will respond better to treatment.

As a Naturopathic physician, a key component of my integrative oncology practice is collaboration with Medical oncologists. I have sent many letters to Medical oncologists with whom I share a patient, informing them of the treatment plan and inviting collaboration. At the very least, this is common professional courtesy and at most, highly beneficial to the patient. Sadly, most do not reply to my letter. I am gratified that a handful of oncologists have replied and we have developed a good relationship. Every Medical oncologist should make an effort to establish a good relationship with a Naturopathic doctor whom they trust. The medical landscape is changing as more and more patients are seeking integrative care. It will serve them well to be directed to a Naturopathic doctor who can collaborate with the Medical oncologist. We need to work together for the benefit of the patient.

Finally, on the subject of "support" throughout the experience of cancer treatment, here are some mental and emotional guidelines for patients. In Western medicine we tend to focus completely on the physical parameters when determining if someone is a suitable candidate for chemotherapy. Before starting something as intense as chemotherapy, it is extremely important that you are mentally prepared for it. Do not go into chemotherapy being fearful of side effects. Patients who are fearful generally do not respond as well to the treatment compared to patients who embrace the chemotherapy.

Whatever treatment that you are doing, you must love the treatment and whole-heartedly embrace it as your answer to this disease. If you are doing radiation then you must learn to love the radiation. If you are doing chemotherapy then you must learn to love the chemotherapy and all the natural supports that you are doing to keep your body strong. By this I mean learn to accept the entire treatment regimen rather than resent it. In other words, embrace the experience with a positive attitude. As difficult as this sounds, remember that our attitudes are a choice. You need to make a substantial effort to mentally prepare for the treatment. It is essential that you are able to whole-heartedly embrace the chemotherapy along with these natural supports as your cure.

In this chapter I discuss the physical supports for chemotherapy but in my opinion these are not nearly as important as the mental/emotional supports that are also required. These mental and emotional supports are described in more detail in chapter 9 (*Intentions and Cancer*). Do not underestimate the importance of being mentally prepared. The physical therapies discussed in this chapter are important because they will give your cells the tools necessary to remain strong during the chemotherapy. You must be proactive about this and feel ready for the treatment mentally and physically.

Omega-3's and Chemotherapy

There is a significant body of evidence that suggests supplementation with omega-3's can help to minimize side effects while increasing the effectiveness of chemotherapy[1]. This potent effect is due to a number of different molecular mechanisms. Supplementation with omega-3's suppresses the expression of COX-2 in tumours, thus decreasing proliferation and angiogenesis in the tumour. It also reduces the activity of genes critical for cancer cells to grow (AP-1, ras, NfKB, bcl-2)[1,2,3,4]. Omega-3's can significantly reduce the side effects from chemotherapy while making the drug more effective through these defined molecular pathways.

A common side effect from chemotherapy is known as "chemo brain" where patients notice a significant decrease in their cognitive capacity and memory[5]. Chemotherapy-induced cognitive impairment is thought to be due to changes to the blood-brain barrier, vascular injury and myelination changes[6]. When patients are supplemented with omega-3's, it can help to reduce the damage to the blood-brain barrier and more effectively regulate the transport of nutrients from the blood to the brain[7].

Chemotherapy is also very oxidative in nature and it can increase the levels of inflammatory markers in the entire body. The systemic inflammation will contribute to many of the symptoms that patients experience[8]. This is similar to having a viral infection. In response to the infection, the immune system releases a significant amount of inflammatory cytokines in an effort to stimulate the immune system and fight the virus. The reason you feel ill during a viral infection often has nothing to do with the virus itself. It is the battle between your immune system and the virus that makes you sick. This systemic inflammation that makes you feel ill during an infection is also present during chemotherapy. Although the source of the inflammatory cytokines is different, the effect is the same. You will not feel great mentally or physically when your body is experiencing systemic inflammation.

Omega-3's are excellent at helping to regulate inflammation while protecting the immune system[9]. It is extremely important that patients take the appropriate dose of omega-3's in order to have positive results. The metabolic demand for these anti-inflammatory molecules will be significantly elevated. I often see patients who are taking self-prescribed omega-3's and the doses are only a fraction of what they should be. The pill forms generally have doses that are simply too low.

Patients on chemotherapy should be taking a minimum of 1900mg of EPA and this is only really attainable when taking a high quality liquid form of omega-3's. The quality of the supplement makes a huge difference and it is necessary to have professional guidance when choosing the proper supplement. In my clinical experience, supplementation with the appropriate dose of omega-3's consistently makes a substantial difference with patients who are experiencing chemo brain.

When cancer progresses, it can often result in patients losing a substantial amount of weight. This is referred to as cachexia and it is commonly seen in late stage cancers. Cancer cells have a high metabolic rate and consequently require a significant amount of energy. At the same time, they are also inefficient because they do not rely on oxygen to supply them with energy. The net result is that cancer cells are wasteful and they burn up the nutrients before healthy cells get the opportunity to utilize them. Omega-3's can be extremely helpful for reversing cachexia even in advanced cases[10,11].

Another important therapeutic effect from omega-3's is their ability to modulate the immune system. When chemotherapy is being administered repeatedly, one of the rate limiting steps is the strength of the immune system. The chemotherapy is very hard on the immune system and you cannot continue therapy if your neutrophil or white blood cell (WBC) count drops below a certain level. Supplementation with omega-3's can help support the immune system and allow it to recover faster from the damage induced by chemotherapy[11,12]. Anything that enables a patient to safely complete additional rounds of chemotherapy with fewer side effects must be regarded as a huge success.

Although there are many positive effects from supplementation with omega-3's, there are some legitimate safety concerns. When used in excess, it can thin the blood and this becomes a concern if the patient is already on blood thinners. It should also not be used shortly before surgery because it will increase the risk of bleeding. These are serious concerns, but when it is used properly under the guidance of a Naturopathic doctor, this is a safe supplement.

Mistletoe Therapy during Chemotherapy

Mistletoe is a parasitic plant that directly derives almost all of its nutrition from other flowering plants. By parasitizing other plants, mistletoe has a competitive advantage over many other forms of life because it does not have to compete for its water and nutrient needs. This description of mistletoe sounds surprisingly similar to how cancer operates. When you look at mistletoe growing on a tree, it looks very much like a tumour. Cancer also gets all of its nutrition from other cells within the human body. This gives it a competitive advantage because it does not abide by the same rules as other cells in the body.

It turns out that mistletoe extracts can be used to effectively treat cancer, even in advanced cases[18,19,20]. In North America this is often considered a "fringe treatment," yet in many European countries, this is a mainstream therapy that is well established by the scientific community. The use of mistletoe dramatically reduces the side effects associated with chemotherapy and radiation. The results are so dramatic that some countries have already made this the standard of care for cancer treatment. The use of mistletoe as the new standard of care reduced medical costs dramatically in these countries because of the significant decrease in complications from chemotherapy and radiation.

Although there are several different ways to administer mistletoe, the most common is regular subcutaneous injections. This involves the use of small insulin needles to inject the mistletoe just under the skin. After injecting the mistletoe lectins, the immune system immediately begins to attack the injected fluid, resulting in a small red rash around the injection site. This immune activation is an excellent outcome in the context of cancer. By activating the immune system at the site of injection, it consequently activates the immune system in the entire body. This helps to protect healthy immune cells during chemotherapy, which ultimately increases the effectiveness of the chemotherapy.

Mistletoe has been shown to stimulate increases in the number and the activity of several types of white blood cells[21]. Immune system enhancing cytokines, such as interleukin-1, interleukin-6, and tumour necrosis factor alpha are released by white blood cells after exposure to mistletoe extracts[22,23]. Other evidence suggests that mistletoe exerts its cytotoxic effects by interfering with protein synthesis in target cells and by inducing apoptosis[24].

Not only is mistletoe well established as an anti-cancer therapy, it significantly improves quality of life when patients are undergoing aggressive cancer therapies. The mechanism for this improved quality of life is not fully understood but it is thought to be due to its influence on the cytokines released by the immune system. I have personally seen patients have dramatic improvements in their quality of life after only a few injections of mistletoe. For optimal effectiveness, the mistletoe should be used as a long-term therapy both during and after chemotherapy.

Mistletoe can also be administered in an IV and there is research to suggest that this can be helpful with painful bone metastasis. IV mistletoe can be a helpful adjunct to IV Vitamin C. Although IV mistletoe is generally well tolerated, it must be administered by an experienced physician. Typically I do not recommend IV mistletoe because it is much more cost effective for patients to administer it subcutaneously. By administering it under the skin, it is easy to monitor how your immune system is reacting to the mistletoe. When mistletoe is given in an IV form, it can be challenging to determine if your immune system is being stimulated or if it has become desensitized to the mistletoe lectins.

Just like any cancer therapy, it is essential that mistletoe is used in the right context. When this therapy is started, there will initially be a swelling of the tumour which is a consequence of the immune activation. The tumour swelling is generally considered a positive change, because it indicates that the immune system is more effectively engaging the tumour. However, if there are any detectable masses contained within the skull, then clearly swelling is not desirable. Mistletoe therapy is contraindicated in patients that have any detectable mass in the brain. It also must be used with caution in patients that are cachexic and malnourished. The sudden release of cytokines associated with immune activation can worsen the malnourished state.

Mistletoe therapy costs less than $200 dollars per month and it can be used in conjunction with other medical therapies. I regularly use mistletoe with my patients at the clinic and it is an effective cancer therapy when used appropriately. On a regular basis, I see patients improve when they use this therapy as part of an integrative cancer plan.

Astragalus and the Immune System

Chemotherapy is toxic to cancer cells but in order to successfully cure cancer you need a functioning immune system. No matter how many rounds of chemotherapy are done, it will not be successful if the immune system is not strong enough to clean up the metabolic mess. When WBC counts start to drop too low, patients will often be prescribed Neupogen to boost the immune system[13]. This drug temporarily elevates WBC levels and reduces the patient's risk of developing an infection. After repeated rounds of chemotherapy, often Neupogen is not enough. The good news is that there are a number of different natural approaches which are effective at supporting the immune system during chemotherapy. Perhaps the most effective natural therapy is astragalus.

Astragalus is an herb that is commonly given to help fight respiratory infections. It is well established in the scientific literature as an immune-boosting supplement that has applications with cancer[14,15]. The mechanism of this immune-boosting effect is poorly defined but the results are undeniable[16]. I have personally witnessed patients who have had an increase in their neutrophil and WBC count during chemotherapy. Their Medical oncologists were shocked to see the numbers improve during such an intense chemotherapy regimen.

Because of its safety and effectiveness, astragalus is regularly used with chemotherapy. It is usually a great way to support the immune system during chemotherapy, but as with any natural supplement, there are exceptions to its use. It is absolutely critical that you have a high quality astragalus supplement. It is not unusual for supplement companies to actually use the wrong part of the plant or have concentrations of astragalosides that are simply insignificant. There are only a select few professional brands that are sufficient in quality to make a difference with the immune system during chemotherapy.

Neuroprotective Therapies

One of the most common side effects from chemotherapy is neuropathy. This is often described as a numbness, tingling or burning in the hands or feet. The damage to the nerves during chemotherapy can be irreversible and it is essential that every patient be proactive in supporting nerve health before any symptoms appear. It is critical that every patient undergoing chemotherapy carefully monitor themselves for signs of neuropathy. If you start to notice numbness or tingling in your hands or feet, you must immediately inform your oncologist so they can modify your dose accordingly. Do not wait for the nurse to tell you that you have signs of neuropathy. If you start to notice changes in your nerves, you must take the initiative to inform the nurse.

Although there are a number of Naturopathic therapies that work well for neuropathy, the ones best supported by scientific evidence are methylcobalamin and benfotiamine (also known as B12 and B1). IV ALA and IV Glutathione are also helpful for preventing the development of neuropathy during chemotherapy. ALA as a nerve support is discussed in more detail in chapter 3 (*Intravenous Therapies and Cancer*). IV Glutathione is a safe adjunctive therapy to the chemotherapy drug oxaliplatin. When given glutathione, patients had fewer side effects (particularly neuropathy) and this did not interfere with the effectiveness of the oxaliplatin[45]. Glutathione is not absorbed orally, therefore it must be administered intravenously. It is critical to recognize that glutathione is safe with some but not all chemotherapies, as it is a potent antioxidant.

Vitamin B12 and B1 are critical for nerve health and it is essential that patients are supported with these nutrients during chemotherapy[17]. Paclitaxel is a chemotherapy commonly given to breast cancer patients and it is notorious for causing substantial neuropathy. This neuropathy is severe and permanent if it is not treated in time. The nerve support should begin before the chemotherapy and it should continue for months after the chemotherapy is complete.

Patients undergoing chemotherapy are usually deficient in B12. If you get a blood test which indicates that B12 levels are high, your cells may still need additional supplementation.

This test simply means that there is sufficient B12 in the blood but it does not indicate whether your body is effectively utilizing the B12. The stress of chemotherapy will significantly impair your body's ability to use the B12. Even if the levels are normal or high, the use of B12 is indicated to support nerve health. I have had many patients who had elevated levels of B12 in their blood but they also had substantial neuropathy. By giving them B12 it helped to significantly improve these symptoms. It is clear that in these cases their cells were not utilizing the B12 even though there was plenty of it in their blood.

B12 can be given sublingually but it is absorbed at high levels when it is administered by an intramuscular injection. These injections (minimum 1mg methylcobalamin) should be done one week after each round of chemotherapy to help minimize the risk of developing neuropathy. Benfotiamine (B1) is given orally as during chemotherapy the metabolic demand for this important vitamin is high. The dose of B1 should be a minimum of 100mg per day to reduce the risk of developing neuropathy. Once the symptoms have started, it can be difficult to reverse the neuropathy. By simply supplementing with these essential vitamins, you can significantly reduce the risk of developing neuropathy in the first place.

Curcumin and Chemotherapy

Turmeric (Curcuma longa) is best known for its spice and it is one of the key components of curry. Curcumin is a substance found in turmeric that is well established as a natural anti-inflammatory[35]. This natural remedy has clearly demonstrated some potent anti-cancer properties in a number of different studies[36,37]. It turns out that this substance fights cancer through a variety of mechanisms without harming non-cancerous cells[36]. Anyone who does a quick Google search will find a significant amount of scientific literature describing the potent anti-cancer effects of curcumin.

Although curcumin is an effective natural therapy, it is generally not safe to use in conjunction with chemotherapy[38]. One of the biggest challenges with integrative oncology is sifting through all the research to determine which natural therapies can be safely used in conjunction with conventional medicine. The goal of these integrative approaches is to support the patient through the conventional toxic procedures while administering natural therapies that have been shown to have positive synergistic effects with the chemotherapy.

There is no doubt that curcumin is effective at preventing and treating cancer when used in the right clinical context. As a general rule it is best to avoid curcumin during chemotherapy because it can protect cancer cells if it is not used properly. There are of course exceptions to this such as with the drug Iressa (Gefitinib) where curcumin definitely increases its effectiveness. Recent research indicates that the anti-cancer effect from curcumin is due to its influence on many different molecular pathways. It seems to powerfully target epidermal growth factor receptor (EGFR) which could explain why it seems to work so well with Iressa[39,40,41]. Another natural remedy that powerfully influences EGFR is milk thistle. Curcumin and milk thistle are a potent combination in circumstances where the primary target is EGFR.

It is essential that curcumin is only given to cancer patients who are under the care of an experienced Naturopathic physician. This is because there are many situations in which curcumin is contraindicated. There are several chemotherapy drugs that will be metabolized more quickly in the presence of curcumin. The net effect is that the chemotherapy is at a therapeutic range for a shorter period of time and the cancer cells are more likely to survive. In these specific circumstances, the chemotherapy is rendered less effective. When used appropriately, curcumin can be a powerful tool to reduce inflammation and it has a number of well documented anti-cancer effects. However, it must be used in the correct clinical context in order to have the desired therapeutic benefit.

Hyperthermia during Chemotherapy

It is a well established fact that cancer cells are vulnerable to heat[25,26]. On a cellular level it makes intuitive sense that cancer cells would be sensitive to heat. Normal cells are spatially arranged so that heat can be distributed evenly and they will not divide if they are physically in contact with adjacent cells. Cancer cells within a tumour will continue to divide regardless of the proximity to adjacent cells. This is one of the hallmarks of cancer. As a result of this uncontrolled growth, the cells in the tumour become densely packed together and this makes it extremely difficult for them to effectively distribute heat.

Hyperthermia treatment is an emerging therapy for patients undergoing chemotherapy and radiation. During these treatments, the patient's core body temperature is artificially raised to mimic a strong fever. This is not a pleasant experience for the patient but it is effective at weakening the cancer cells. It makes the cancer cells more vulnerable to chemotherapy and radiation. It is important to note that this is very different than an infrared sauna. An infrared sauna can be helpful as a gentle detoxification, but it will certainly not raise the core body temperature enough to weaken the cancer cells. A true hyperthermia device raises the core body temperature so significantly that the patient must be medically supervised during the treatment.

More advanced devices are now available which only heat up the local environment of the tumour. This is more comfortable for the patient, making it possible to heat up the tumour much more than is possible with the whole body hyperthermia. Whole body hyperthermia devices raise the core body temperature to approximately 40°C and this slow process takes approximately 3-4 hours. With loco-regional hyperthermia, it is possible to increase the temperature of the tumour well beyond 40°C and the process is much shorter. Hyperthermia is probably the most potent chemo and radio sensitizing method currently known.

When any cell is exposed to heat, immediate biochemical and genetic changes occur so that the cell can adapt to the new warmer environment. One of the most potent responses that allows these cells to survive the heat is the production of heat shock proteins (HSP)[27]. These HSPs protect components within the cell that are vulnerable to heat damage. Currently there is a major push with pharmaceutical companies to develop drugs that inhibit these proteins.

There are several natural compounds which act as potent heat shock protein inhibitors. These substances are only safe when used in the right clinical context and you need to consult a Naturopathic doctor to know if this is the best therapy for your specific type of cancer. One example is quercetin, which is a bioflavonoid that is well documented as a powerful inhibitor of heat shock proteins in cancer cells[28,29,30,31,32,33].

Cancer cells are naturally vulnerable to heat because of how densely the cells are packed together. When hyperthermia is combined with quercetin, the results are dramatic[34]. One study on prostate carcinoma concluded that:

> When combined in a treatment protocol with hyperthermia, quercetin drastically inhibited tumour growth and potently amplified the effects of hyperthermia on two prostate tumour types, PC-3 and DU-145 *in vivo*. These experiments, thus, suggest the use of quercetin as a hyperthermia sensitizer in the treatment of prostate carcinoma. (Asea et al. 354)

It is critical to point out two things. Firstly, quercetin is safe with most but not all chemotherapy drugs and you need professional guidance to know if this is safe for you. Secondly, the quality of the quercetin supplement makes a big difference. Generally speaking, quercetin is very poorly absorbed and there are only a few professional brands of sufficient quality that are effective at sensitizing the cancer cells. In some cases, intravenous quercetin is more appropriate but this must be performed by an experienced physician because there is a high risk of a hypersensitivity reaction when administered intravenously.

The mainstream medical community is changing its tune with regard to hyperthermia. In private hospitals in the United States, it is commonly used because it is so effective. In Canada, there are only a handful of clinics that currently offer this therapy. I am very proud of the fact that Yaletown Naturopathic Clinic has one of the most advanced loco-regional hyperthermia devices in North America. These devices are safe and effective when used appropriately. As the evidence for this therapy accumulates, in the near future hyperthermia combined with these natural approaches will undoubtedly become the standard of care for cancer patients.

Other Common Chemotherapy Supports

The therapies described in this chapter are certainly not the only supports available. There are many other natural supplements that can be helpful in supporting patients through chemotherapy. You have to be careful about the things that you put into your body as there are many potential interactions with chemotherapy. With the guidance of an experienced Naturopathic physician, you can develop a plan that is truly tailored to your unique concerns. The specific chemotherapy supports used will vary significantly depending on the drugs used and the unique health concerns of the patient.

Vitamin D can also be an effective chemotherapy support in some circumstances. A common chemotherapy protocol is the combination of carboplatin and paclitaxel. It is well documented that carboplatin rapidly depletes the body of Vitamin D. The other drug in this protocol, paclitaxel, has been shown to be more effective when patients are supplemented with Vitamin D. It is obvious based on this information that patients on this protocol should be supplemented with Vitamin D. For optimal effects, it is critical that patients are supplied with the proper dose of Vitamin D. Due to the fact that it is fat soluble, obese patients will need higher doses to reach therapeutic levels. Unfortunately Vitamin D is rarely recommended which is a shame because patients need professional guidance with the dosing. It is not beneficial to be on super high doses of this fat soluble vitamin but it is helpful when patients are given the proper therapeutic dose.

There is no doubt that chemotherapy is toxic to both cancerous and healthy cells. Some patients upon reading that chemotherapy is toxic decide to initiate a detoxification protocol while on chemotherapy. That is the absolute worst time to do a detoxification. When your body is put through a detoxification protocol, this is initially very stressful on your cells. It results in a significant amount of toxins being mobilized which is stressful on the liver and kidneys. These detox protocols can certainly be used to promote general wellness when they are used properly. However, they should not be used while the body is acutely stressed with something else such as chemotherapy. Wait at least three weeks post chemotherapy before initiating any detox protocol.

Oral Mucositis

One of the most uncomfortable side effects from chemotherapy (and in some cases of radiation) is oral mucositis. These are open wounds in the mouth that are painful and they are slow to heal due to the presence of chemotherapy. The most uncomfortable ulcerations are in the oral cavity but the reality is that these wounds can occur anywhere throughout the gastrointestinal tract. Generally this side effect tends to occur during the first few rounds of chemotherapy. It is rare for this side effect to occur during the later rounds.

Conventional medicine has little to offer when it comes to controlling the oral mucositis. However, there are several natural therapies which can help patients heal from this painful side effect. One of the most simple and effective remedies is cabbage juice. Buy yourself a juicer and use it to break down the cabbage into a smoothie. Cabbage contains nutrients that help to heal these wounds throughout the gastrointestinal tract. It is thought that the glutamine content of the cabbage is the primary ingredient responsible for this effect, but it is clear that there is much more to cabbage than simply glutamine. I have observed in a clinical setting on several occasions where glutamine had no effect on the wounds, but when the patient used cabbage juice the wounds healed incredibly fast.

Another common remedy used to heal wounds in the mouth is honey. Many patients avoid honey due to the high sugar content. Generally speaking, it would be advisable to limit your intake of honey because it is rich in sugar. However, when used moderately it can be helpful for oral mucositis. The benefits of using honey in these situations far outweighs the risks.

Recently there was an interesting study from Italy in a mainstream oncology journal regarding the use of coffee and honey to prevent oral mucositis during chemotherapy. Patients who regularly consumed coffee and honey were much less likely to get oral mucositis, and those who did get it had less severe mucositis[46]. What is interesting about this study is that the coffee that was used was inexpensive instant coffee. This does not mean that only instant coffee would be effective, but it is interesting to note that it does not have to be high quality coffee to have the desired effect.

These natural approaches to oral mucositis should be used as soon as there is any sign of inflammation in the mouth. It is challenging to heal any wound when a patient is undergoing chemotherapy. This is why surgery cannot be done until six weeks after chemotherapy is completed. The body's ability to heal wounds is severely impaired from these medications. It is for this reason that you must address the concern before it manifests into a significant problem. As soon as there is any indication of a wound developing in the mouth, you must address this concern rapidly and aggressively.

Nausea and Vomiting

One of the most common side effects from chemotherapy is nausea. Patients are generally prescribed anti-nausea medication before initiating chemotherapy because it is reasonable to expect that they will experience this side effect. The most commonly prescribed medication for nausea is metclopramide. This is a dopamine antagonist that can significantly reduce nausea and vomiting. Although it is generally quite effective, it certainly doesn't work for everyone and many patients are left looking for an alternative solution to this uncomfortable side effect.

There are many different metabolic pathways that can lead to the sensation of nausea. Metclopramide only targets one of these pathways and it will not be effective if the nausea is due to the stimulation of a different metabolic pathway. One effective prescription for nausea is a cream composed of three different medications: diphenhydramine (Benadryl), dexamethasone and metclopramide. These medications are absorbed through the skin and the effects are almost immediate. The reason it is so effective is that each component of this cream targets a completely different pathway linked to nausea. One major benefit of this topical approach is that when the main symptom is nausea, obviously swallowing pills is challenging. In extreme cases, even the thought of swallowing a pill would trigger a strong bout of nausea. Using a cream bypasses the need for the pills and you still get the positive effect from these conventional medications.

There is evidence to suggest that cannaboids can be helpful in patients with drug resistant nausea because they gently influence several pathways that inhibit nausea. Many patients immediately resort to cannaboids to assist with the nausea but there are other options which are easier and more effective. The most common and, in my opinion, the most effective natural anti-nausea remedy is ginger.

Ginger inhibits nausea by a completely different mechanism. It is a potent 5-HT3 antagonist, which means that it inhibits the activity of serotonin. Serotonin is a neurotransmitter that also is strongly linked to nausea and vomiting. A strong ginger tea can often make a profound difference in patients that have stopped responding to conventional medications. The ginger does not have to be taken in replacement of conventional anti-nausea medications. In fact, it works best if taken with conventional medications because then you have multiple pathways being inhibited rather than just one.

It is easy to make the ginger tea. Just go to your local grocery store and buy some fresh ginger root. Cut the ginger into small pieces until you have a handful of ginger slices, then place the ginger into a pot of boiling water. Let it simmer for 15 minutes with the lid on to keep all the volatile oils contained within the tea. Filter the pieces of ginger out of the tea using a strainer and allow the tea to cool until it is a pleasant warm tea. Slowly sip at the tea and give it about 30 minutes to work. Some people find the tea more tolerable if honey is added after the ginger pieces have been filtered out.

Metronomic Chemotherapy

Most patients in North America are given the highest dose of chemotherapy possible in an effort to kill the cancerous cells. The logic is that when you give a higher dose it will kill more cancer cells. This is a true statement and it makes sense. When you surround cancer cells with a greater concentration of chemotherapy, then more cells are likely to die.

There is however a fundamental problem with this approach. Just as the drugs are toxic to cancer cells, they are also toxic to healthy cells. As a result it is not possible to give continuous treatments at these high doses. It is necessary to give the body breaks between rounds of chemotherapy so that the body and the immune system can recover from exposure to these toxins. The problem is that during these breaks the cancer also has time to recover. Not only does it have time to recover, but the cancerous cells that remain are more likely to be resistant to the next round of chemotherapy.

There is a solution to this problem called metronomic chemotherapy. Essentially this involves the use of much lower doses of chemotherapy with much shorter breaks between rounds. In some cases there are no breaks in between and it involves continuous low dose chemotherapy. It appears that at low doses the chemotherapy has a profound anti-angiogenic effect[42]. Tumours need a constant supply of blood to sustain their rapid growth. At low doses, the chemotherapy appears to significantly impair the tumours ability to develop new blood vessels.

The anti-angiogenic effect of metronomic chemotherapy significantly enhances the effect of anti-vascular agents such as Avastin[44]. This synergy is part of an exciting new field of research that has significant implications for many different solid tumours. This is a treatment option for tumours that would otherwise not respond effectively to the typical anti-vascular agents.

Obviously when the chemotherapy is administered at low doses there is a significant reduction in side effects. The immune system does not become nearly as depleted when it is exposed to these lower doses. This allows the body to maintain a high level of anti-tumour activity during the course of treatment, making metronomic chemotherapy a much more desirable option for many patients.

Recent evidence also suggests that the cancerous cells are less likely to develop resistance to chemotherapy when they are exposed to continuous low doses[43]. At these lower doses, there is less of a selective pressure for the cancer cells to develop resistance. The dose however is high enough that it is able to suppress the growth of tumours. Treating cancer in this way changes how we perceive the disease. It shifts the treatment mentality from being a lethal disease which must be treated aggressively to a chronic disease that can be managed and stabilized.

It is interesting to see the differences in how cancer is treated across the world. In Europe, metronomic chemotherapy is commonly used for many different types of cancer. It is better tolerated by patients and the immune system remains strong. The tumours are less likely to become resistant to the drug and it significantly slows the growth of cancerous cells. Metronomic chemotherapy is also cost effective because it uses low doses of standard chemotherapy drugs that have a long history of use.

In North America, the use of metronomic chemotherapy is rare. There seems to be a strong emphasis on the newer and more expensive targeted drugs. It appears that the resistance to metronomic chemotherapy in North America is due to the financially motivated pharmaceutical companies and it has nothing to do with the effectiveness of the drug. These companies certainly prefer oncologists to use new expensive drugs rather than older and inexpensive drugs to be used at low doses. It is unfortunate that finances are dictating the standard of care when there is such a simple cost effective option available for many patients.

Although these targeted drugs are exciting and they represent a new era of cancer treatment, they are not the only drugs that can fight cancer. We should not just blindly abandon older chemotherapy drugs in favour of newer, more expensive drugs. Rather, we should make an effort to improve existing chemotherapy protocols, such as using the metronomic approach. This will not only benefit patients; it will also benefit the economy when these inexpensive (and in some cases more effective) drugs are used.

Summary:

- Omega-3's help to reduce inflammation and support the immune system

- Astragalus can be used to boost the immune system and maintain WBC count during chemotherapy

- Benfotiamine (Vitamin B1) is helpful to support nerve health and prevent neuropathy

- Methylcobalamin (Vitamin B12) as an intramuscular injection one week after each round of chemotherapy preserves nerve health

- IV ALA and IV Glutathione can be neuroprotective when used with certain chemotherapies

- Mistletoe should be administered subcutaneously to support the immune system and reduce side effects of chemotherapy and radiation

- Fasting 48 hours before chemotherapy and 24 hours afterwards (See chapter 2 on *Diet and Cancer)* can reduce side effects while increasing effectiveness of chemotherapy

- Hyperthermia immediately following infusion of chemotherapy can enhance the effectiveness of chemotherapy

- Avoid curcumin and quercetin unless under the supervision of a Naturopathic physician

- Ginger tea can effectively address chemotherapy-induced nausea

- Honey, coffee and cabbage juice can help to heal oral mucositis

References:

1. Hardman, W. Elaine. "Omega-3 fatty acids to augment cancer therapy." *The Journal of Nutrition* 132.11 (2002): 3508S-3512S.

2. Sawyer, Michael B., and Catherine J. Field. "Possible Mechanisms of ω-3 PUFA Anti-tumour Action." Dietary omega-3 polyunsaturated fatty acids and cancer. Springer Netherlands, 2010. 3-38.

3. Kang, Jing X., and Karsten H. Weylandt. "Modulation of inflammatory cytokines by omega-3 fatty acids." Lipids in Health and Disease. Springer Netherlands, 2008. 133-143.

4. Chen, Z. Y., and N. W. Istfan. "Docosahexaenoic acid is a potent inducer of apoptosis in HT-29 colon cancer cells." *Prostaglandins, leukotrienes and essential fatty acids* 63.5 (2000): 301-308.

5. Staat, Kari, and Milena Segatore. "The phenomenon of chemo brain." *Clinical journal of Oncology Nursing* 9.6 (2005): 713-721.

6. Evens, Katrina, and Valerie S. Eschiti. "Cognitive effects of cancer treatment:" chemo brain" explained." *Clinical Journal of Oncology Nursing* 13.6 (2009): 661-666.

7. Pifferi, F., et al. "n-3 Fatty acids modulate brain glucose transport in endothelial cells of the blood–brain barrier." *Prostaglandins, Leukotrienes and Essential Fatty Acids* 77.5 (2007): 279-286.

8. Mills, Paul J., et al. "The relationship between fatigue and quality of life and inflammation during anthracycline-based chemotherapy in breast cancer." *Biological Psychology* 69.1 (2005): 85-96.

9. Simopoulos, Artemis P. "Omega-3 fatty acids in inflammation and autoimmune diseases." *Journal of the American College of Nutrition* 21.6 (2002): 495-505.

10. Deans, Christopher, and Stephen J. Wigmore. "Systemic inflammation, cachexia and prognosis in patients with cancer." Current Opinion in *Clinical Nutrition & Metabolic Care* 8.3 (2005): 265-269.

11. Gogos, Charalambos A., et al. "Dietary omega-3 polyunsaturated fatty acids plus vitamin E restore immunodeficiency and prolong survival for severely ill patients with generalized malignancy." *Cancer* 82.2 (1998): 395-402.

12. Berquin, Isabelle M., Iris J. Edwards, and Yong Q. Chen. "Multi-targeted therapy of cancer by omega-3 fatty acids." *Cancer letters* 269.2 (2008): 363-377.

13. Vogel, Charles L., et al. "First and subsequent cycle use of pegfilgrastim prevents febrile neutropenia in patients with breast cancer: a multicenter, double-blind, placebo-controlled phase III study." *Journal of Clinical Oncology* 23.6 (2005): 1178-1184.

14. Block, Keith I., and Mark N. Mead. "Immune system effects of echinacea, ginseng, and astragalus: a review." *Integrative Cancer Therapies* 2.3 (2003): 247-267.

15. Chu, Da-Tong, et al. "Fractionated extract of Astragalus membranaceus, a Chinese medicinal herb, potentiates LAK cell cytotoxicity generated by a low dose of recombinant interleukin-2." *Journal of clinical & laboratory immunology* 26.4 (1988): 183-187.

16. Ríos, José-Luis. "Effects of triterpenes on the immune system." *Journal of ethnopharmacology* 128.1 (2010): 1-14.

17. Dizaye, Kawa F., and Chro Y. Qadir. "Effects of Benfotiamine and Methylcobalamin on Paclitaxel induced Peripheral neuropathy." *Middle East Journal of Internal Medicine* 7.1 (2014).

18. Murray, Michael T. The healing power of herbs: the enlightened person's guide to the wonders of medicinal plants. Rev. 1995. 253-9.

19. Samtleben, Rainer, et al. "Mistletoe lectins as immunostimulants (chemistry, pharmacology and clinic)." *Immunomodulatory Agents from Plants.* Birkhäuser Basel, 1999. 223-241.

20. Hajto, T., and Ch Lanzrein. "Natural killer and antibody-dependent cell-mediated cytotoxicity activities and large granular lymphocyte frequencies in Viscum album-treated breast cancer patients." *Oncology* 43.2 (1986): 93-97.

21. Büssing, A., A. Regnery, and K. Schweizer. "Effects of Viscum album L. on cyclophosphamide-treated peripheral blood mononuclear cells in vitro: sister chromatid exchanges and activation/proliferation marker expression." *Cancer letters* 94.2 (1995): 199-205.

22. Hajto, Tibor. "Immunomodulatory effects of Iscador: a Viscum album preparation." *Oncology* 43.Suppl. 1 (1986): 51-65.

23. Hajto T, Hostanska K, Frei K, et al.: Increased secretion of tumor necrosis factors alpha, interleukin 1, and interleukin 6 by human mononuclear cells exposed to beta-galactoside-specific lectin from clinically applied mistletoe extract. Cancer Res 50 (11): 3322-6, 1990.

24. Mengs, U., et al. "Antitumoral effects of an intravesically applied aqueous mistletoe extract on urinary bladder carcinoma MB49 in mice." *Anticancer research* 20.5B (1999): 3565-3568.

25. van der Zee, Jill. "Heating the patient: a promising approach?." *Annals of oncology* 13.8 (2002): 1173-1184..

26. van der Zee, Jill. "Hyperthermia in addition to radiotherapy." *Clinical Oncology* 19.3 (2007): S18.

27. De Maio, Antonio. "Heat shock proteins: facts, thoughts, and dreams." *Shock* 11.1 (1999): 1-12.

28. Hansen, R. K., et al. "Quercetin inhibits heat shock protein induction but not heat shock factor DNA-binding in human breast carcinoma cells." Biochemical and biophysical research communications 239.3 (1997): 851-856.

29. Gonzalez, Oscar, et al. "The heat shock protein inhibitor Quercetin attenuates hepatitis C virus production." *Hepatology* 50.6 (2009): 1756-1764.

30. Wei, Yu-quan, et al. "Induction of apoptosis by quercetin: involvement of heat shock protein." *Cancer Research* 54.18 (1994): 4952-4957.

31. Zanini, Cristina, et al. "Inhibition of heat shock proteins (HSP) expression by quercetin and differential doxorubicin sensitization in neuroblastoma and Ewing's sarcoma cell lines." *Journal of neurochemistry* 103.4 (2007): 1344-1354.

32. Hosokawa, Nobuko, et al. "Flavonoids inhibit the expression of heat shock proteins." *Cell structure and function* 15.6 (1990): 393-401.

33. Elia, Guiliano, and M. G. Santoro. "Regulation of heat shock protein synthesis by quercetin in human erythroleukaemia cells." *Biochem. J* 300 (1994): 201-209.

34. Asea, A., et al. "Effects of the flavonoid drug quercetin on the response of human prostate tumours to hyperthermia in vitro and in vivo." *International journal of hyperthermia* 17.4 (2001): 347-356.

35. Satoskar, R. R., S. J. Shah, and S. G. Shenoy. "Evaluation of anti-inflammatory property of curcumin (diferuloyl methane) in patients with postoperative inflammation." *International journal of clinical pharmacology, therapy, and toxicology* 24.12 (1986): 651-654.

36. Ravindran, Jayaraj, Sahdeo Prasad, and Bharat B. Aggarwal. "Curcumin and cancer cells: how many ways can curry kill tumor cells selectively?." *The AAPS journal* 11.3 (2009): 495-510.

37. Dhillon, Navneet, et al. "Phase II trial of curcumin in patients with advanced pancreatic cancer." *Clinical Cancer Research* 14.14 (2008): 4491-4499.

38. Somasundaram, Sivagurunathan, et al. "Dietary curcumin inhibits chemotherapy-induced apoptosis in models of human breast cancer." *Cancer research* 62.13 (2002): 3868-3875.

39. Shukla, Yogeshwer, Annu Arora, and Pankaj Taneja. "Antimutagenic potential of curcumin on chromosomal aberrations in Wistar rats." Mutation *Research/Genetic Toxicology and Environmental Mutagenesis* 515.1 (2002): 197-202.

40. Lee, Jen-Yi, et al. "Curcumin induces EGFR degradation in lung adeno-carcinoma and modulates p38 activation in intestine: the versatile adjuvant for gefitinib therapy." PloS one 6.8 (2011): e23756.

41. Patel, Bhaumik B., et al. "Curcumin targets FOLFOX-surviving colon cancer cells via inhibition of EGFRs and IGF-1R." *Anticancer Research* 30.2 (2010): 319-325.

42. Kerbel, Robert S., and Barton A. Kamen. "The anti-angiogenic basis of metronomic chemotherapy." *Nature Reviews Cancer* 4.6 (2004): 423-436.

43. Kareva, Irina, David J. Waxman, and Giannoula Lakka Klement. "Metronomic chemotherapy: An attractive alternative to maximum tolerated dose therapy that can activate anti-tumor immunity and minimize therapeutic resistance." *Cancer letters* (2014).

44. Montagna, Emilia, et al. "Metronomic chemotherapy combined with bevacizumab and erlotinib in patients with metastatic HER2-negative breast cancer: clinical and biological activity." *Clinical breast cancer* 12.3 (2012): 207-214.

45. Cascinu, Stefano, et al. "Neuroprotective effect of reduced glutathione on oxaliplatin-based chemotherapy in advanced colorectal cancer: a randomized, double-blind, placebo-controlled trial." *Journal of Clinical Oncology* 20.16 (2002): 3478-3483.

46. Holt, S. "Honey/coffee product may reduce chemotherapy-induced oral mucositis." *Focus on Alternative and Complementary Therapies* 19.4 (2014): 225-226.

Chemotherapy Support

Chapter 5

Radiation Support

**"Natural forces within us are
the true healers of disease."
- Hippocrates**

It is fascinating to see how our understanding of radiation
has evolved over the last 50 years. My grandfather told me
that when he was young, people shopping for shoes would
put their feet in an X-ray device so that they could determine
if their shoe size was correct. The amount of radiation from
these older devices was significant and obviously these would
never be used now, given our understanding of radiation.

Although I knew radiation was something that should be
avoided, it was not until high school that I understood the
effects radiation can have on the body. My high school physics
teacher was undergoing radiation therapy on his skull. He did
not reveal the diagnosis, but he thought that this would be

a good opportunity to explain the physics behind radiation. At first I was shocked that someone could receive radiation to their brain with seemingly no side effects. As his treatments continued, he started to lose hair and his fatigue became obvious. At the time I had no interest in radiation, but his lecture was one that I will never forget. I could never have predicted at that point in time that I would enter a career working with cancer, but this simple lecture was certainly one of the experiences in my life that led me down this path.

Radiation has been used for decades as one of the primary conventional cancer therapies. Although radiation can be an effective option, it also has potential for significant side effects including burns and permanent tissue damage. Often the radiation doses are spread out over the course of several days or weeks. Generally speaking, if the target area for the radiation is small (such as a localized tumour), then the side effects tend to be quite manageable. When the target area is large, the radiation dose must be increased and the risk for side effects increases dramatically. The good news is that there are several natural therapies which can be used to decrease side effects and increase the effectiveness of radiation therapy.

Oxygen is abundant in every cell in the body and radiation interacts with oxygen to create high-energy free radicals which damage the DNA. The goal is to damage the DNA within the cancer cells so significantly that they are unable to recover. The targeted abnormal cells will then die as a consequence of the DNA damage. The concern with radiation is that during this procedure, healthy cells will also be radiated, thus indiscriminately damaging their DNA. This has potential to create new cancerous cells in the body which often takes many years to develop into a clinical disease.

There are many different types of radiation therapy and the clinical picture determines the course of treatment. The goal of radiation therapy is to deliver the maximum radiation dose possible to cancerous cells while minimizing contact with healthy cells. Any cell that is exposed to radiation can be permanently altered in its growth pattern. Cells that divide rapidly are more vulnerable to radiation than cells that grow slowly.

When radiation is unsuccessful, it is often due to what is known as the hypoxic cell problem. Radiation is simply not as effective in cellular environments that are low in oxygen. One of the hallmarks of cancer is that it is capable of generating energy without oxygen. If you think about the structure of a tumour, it is a disorganized densely packed mass of cells. There is a poor supply of blood to these tissues and it is difficult for oxygen to penetrate deeply into the core of the tumour. Cancer cells within tumours have evolved to survive in oxygen poor environments.

This evolutionary adaptation makes cancer cells deep within the tumour resistant to radiation. The radiation beam is simply not able to generate the same amount of damaging oxygen free radicals within these cells. There are several natural compounds which can be used to circumvent this hypoxic cell problem. Many of these natural therapies also have the added benefit of controlling the inflammation that can become quite severe after multiple treatments of radiation.

Regardless of the type of radiation therapy used or the location of the target area, the supportive therapies tend to be similar. The molecular targets and rationale for treatment remain the same despite any variations in the therapy. As with any treatment plan, it should be specifically tailored to that individual and these subtle changes to the treatment plan will require clinical expertise.

The most potent natural radio-sensitizer is without a doubt niacin—also known as Vitamin B3 or niacinamide. This simple natural compound is well established as a vasodilator. In other words, it increases the blood supply to the tumour which increases the concentration of oxygen within the tumour. This makes the cancer cells deep within the tumour much more vulnerable to radiation[1,2,3]. Niacinamide is safe to take throughout radiation and patients should take at least 500mg three times per day during radiation. Some pharmacists will warn patients about the "niacin flush" which is a common symptom at high doses of niacin. Basically it causes flushing of the face and this can cause some discomfort in extreme cases. In reality, if you are taking a high quality niacinamide supplement that has sustained release, then the flushing should be a non issue. If you are taking high doses that are causing your face to flush due to the vasodilation, then chances are that the tumour is also experiencing that same vasodilatory effect.

Another critical radiation support (especially in cases of head and neck cancers) is zinc[9]. Several clinical trials have demonstrated that supplementation with zinc significantly reduces side effects from radiation including mucositis and dermatitis. One common side effect from radiation is loss of taste which can lead to weight loss because this translates into a significantly diminished appetite. Zinc is extremely helpful at preventing and in some cases reversing the loss of taste that results from radiation[11,12]. Generally speaking, zinc is well tolerated and patients should take approximately 60mg per day with meals during radiation. There are several different forms of zinc and they differ substantially in their bioavailability. The form that I typically recommend is zinc picolinate due to its optimal absorption.

Curcumin is another natural therapy which helps to sensitize cancer cells to radiation. It is a potent anti-inflammatory agent that can reduce complications associated with high doses of radiation. Curcumin is a potent inhibitor of a protein called nuclear factor kappa beta (NfKb) and of cyclooxygenase-2[13,14].

This inhibition reduces local inflammation around the tumour while making it more vulnerable to the radiation. Curcumin is poorly absorbed so it is critical that patients use a high quality supplement. There are a handful of professional brands which are well absorbed. A Naturopathic physician skilled in oncology can help you choose the most effective supplement.

Omega-3's can also be helpful to reduce the inflammation associated with radiation. Patients often feel better mentally and physically when they are well supported by omega-3's during radiation. There are however, some potential interactions with omega-3 supplementation and blood thinners. At higher doses, the omega-3's can thin the blood, although this effect is minor when compared to blood thinners such as warfarin. If you are on warfarin during radiation, talk to your physician about switching to heparin. Warfarin does not improve clinical response to radiation therapy (or chemotherapy) as much as the anticoagulant heparin[15].

It is extremely important that every patient undergoing radiation therapy strictly avoid oil-based medicines on the skin. The radiation beam will interact with the oil and it will cause severe burns. Putting oil on your skin and washing it off before the treatment is not sufficient. It is not possible to wash off enough of the oil to prevent burns. This is information your radiation oncologist should give you. Unfortunately, I have personally witnessed several cases where patients were not informed of this and they experienced severe burns as a result. It is not worth the risk. If you are doing radiation therapy, you should strictly avoid all oil-based creams.

Aloe vera can be very helpful to promote healing of radiation burns after the radiation therapy is complete. The aloe vera gel derived directly from the plant can be safely applied during radiation therapy. It can also be taken orally during radiation, but you cannot apply any aloe vera creams or oils topically until all the radiation treatments are complete[16]. This simple therapy has been used for centuries and there is no doubt that it is helpful for healing burns and wounds.

It is true that high doses of antioxidants are contraindicated during radiation therapy[10]. Patients should avoid high levels of synthetic antioxidants, but it is completely safe to get antioxidants from your food. In fact, radiation creates so much oxidative damage that patients should be encouraged to consume antioxidant-rich foods. The antioxidants in fruits such as blueberries and blackberries are not sufficient to interfere with the radiation, but it is sufficient to help protect healthy cells from the effects of radiation. It is often described in the literature as one step back and two steps forward. The net result is a step in the right direction!

The most important dietary change for patients to make during radiation is a low glycemic diet. Often radiation oncologists will state that diet does not make a difference and that patients should eat whatever they want. This is simply not true, and their own medical journals clearly state that diet can make a big difference in quality of life and influence clinical outcomes[4,5,6,7,8]. When looking at the literature, one common theme that emerges is that patients with a reduced intake of sugar respond better to radiation than patients who consume more sugar. In some of these studies, the positive effects are attributed to the ketogenic diet which is high in fat and low in sugar. The ketogenic diet is certainly indicated for brain tumours undergoing radiation therapy. However, in most cases simply avoiding sugar is sufficient.

I regularly hear from patients that the most common beverages in the radiation therapy waiting room are sugar rich soda drinks. This is outrageous given what we know about the interaction between sugar and cancer. Every patient should be actively encouraged to eat healthy and avoid foods that we know are harmful.

Hyperthermia and Radiation

Hyperthermia is the application of heat to cancerous cells. This is very different from an infrared sauna. A hyperthermia machine is an advanced medical device that heats up the cancerous tissue significantly, and the patients must be medically monitored throughout the procedure. More recently, hyperthermia has emerged as an effective treatment to sensitize tumours to radiation therapy[17,18,19]. In Germany, these therapies are common and they are used in a hospital setting. In North America, it seems that this therapy is not commonly used despite the growing body of irrefutable evidence. Hyperthermia is not meant to be used as a stand alone therapy. It is intended as an adjunctive cancer therapy that improves outcomes when combined with chemotherapy or radiation.

Hyperthermia alters the blood supply within the tumour to make it more susceptible to radiation[19]. The heat also triggers cell death pathways in the cancerous cells. The chaotic structure of the densely packed tumour makes the cancer cells within the tumour vulnerable to heat. These cells are inefficient at distributing heat and their poor vascular supply allows them to remain resistant to radiation. The heat from the hyperthermia device increases the blood flow to the tumour which allows the radiation to act more effectively at the tumour site. There are many well controlled clinical trials which clearly show that radiation is more effective when it is combined with localized hyperthermia.

Ideally you want to have the hyperthermia treatment immediately after the radiation is complete. This allows the radiation to take advantage of the metabolic changes that occur when the tumour mass is heated. Unfortunately, in North America there are very few centres which offer this therapy. The clinic that I work at, Yaletown Naturopathic Clinic, has an advanced loco-regional hyperthermia device. Localized hyperthermia is an effective adjunctive therapy to radiation when used appropriately. In my opinion this is a therapy that every patient undergoing chemotherapy or radiation should use.

Post Radiation Damage

It is not uncommon to have a delayed negative reaction to radiation. I have personally witnessed on several occasions where patients tolerated the radiation well but years later complications started to arise. The delayed post-radiation damage is often due to the chronic low-grade inflammation at the sites of radiation. This constant low-grade inflammation results in the accumulation of scar tissue and damage to the microvasculature. This is another reason why it is critical to continue supporting patients naturally long after the treatment is complete.

One of the most common sites for patients to experience this delayed radiation damage is in the anal sphincter. When radiation is used on such a delicate structure, there is always a risk of damage. It is not unusual for patients to have no problems controlling their bowel movements for years after getting radiation to the anal sphincter. Then suddenly, several years after radiation, they are no longer able to control their bowel movements. This same phenomenon can also occur in patients who received radiation on the prostate. They can suddenly have erectile dysfunction years after receiving radiation. It is important to point out that this is less common with the more advanced radiation techniques that are now used on the prostate.

The bottom line is that the effects from radiation can occur years after the procedure, so it is critical that patients continue to have integrative support long after radiation is complete. By supporting patients after chemotherapy and radiation, it is possible to reduce the risk of future complications. Regularly following up with a Naturopathic doctor makes it more likely that these complications will be identified before they become a serious concern.

Summary:

- Niacinamide when used prior to radiation increases blood flow to the tumour
- Zinc picolinate enhances the effectiveness of radiation and reduces side effects
- Curcumin can help reduce the inflammation associated with radiation
- Omega-3's can significantly reduce inflammation and support the immune system during radiation
- Do not use any oil-based creams on your skin before or during radiation therapy
- Aloe vera can help with burns only after radiation therapy is complete
- Localized hyperthermia treatments enhance the effectiveness of the radiation

References:

1. Kjellén, Elisabeth, et al. "Effect of hyperthermia and/or nicotinamide on the radiation response of a C3H mammary carcinoma." *European Journal of Cancer and Clinical Oncology* 25.12 (1989): 1733-1737.

2. Stratford, Michael RL, and Madeleine F. Dennis. "Pharmacokinetics and biochemistry studies on nicotinamide in the mouse." *Cancer chemotherapy and pharmacology* 34.5 (1994): 399-404.

3. Horsman, Michael R. "Nicotinamide and other benzamide analogs as agents for overcoming hypoxic cell radiation resistance in tumours." *Acta Oncologica* 34.5 (1995): 571-587.

4. Isenring, Elisabeth A., Sandra Capra, and Judith D. Bauer. "Nutrition intervention is beneficial in oncology outpatients receiving radiotherapy to the gastrointestinal or head and neck area." *British Journal of Cancer* 91.3 (2004): 447-452.

5. Abdelwahab, Mohammed G., et al. "The ketogenic diet is an effective adjuvant to radiation therapy for the treatment of malignant glioma." *PloS one* 7.5 (2012): e36197.

6. Piquet, Marie-Astrid, et al. "Early nutritional intervention in oropharyngeal cancer patients undergoing radiotherapy." *Supportive care in cancer* 10.6 (2002): 502-504.

7. Klimberg, V. Suzanne, et al. "Prophylactic glutamine protects the intestinal mucosa from radiation injury." *Cancer* 66.1 (1990): 62-68.

8. Bounous, G., et al. "Dietary protection during radiation therapy." *Strahlentherapie* 149.5 (1975): 476-483.

9. Lin, Li-Ching, et al. "Zinc supplementation to improve mucositis and dermatitis in patients after radiotherapy for head-and-neck cancers: a double-blind, randomized study." *International Journal of Radiation Oncology* Biology* Physics* 65.3 (2006): 745-750.

10. Lawenda, Brian D., et al. "Should supplemental antioxidant administration be avoided during chemotherapy and radiation therapy?." *Journal of the national cancer institute* 100.11 (2008): 773-783.

11. Mossman, Kenneth L., and Robert I. Henkin. "Radiation-induced changes in taste acuity in cancer patients." *International Journal of Radiation Oncology* Biology* Physics* 4.7 (1978): 663-670.

12. Ripamonti, Carla, et al. "A randomized, controlled clinical trial to evaluate the effects of zinc sulfate on cancer patients with taste alterations caused by head and neck irradiation." *Cancer* 82.10 (1998): 1938-1945.

13. Dhillon, Navneet, et al. "Phase II trial of curcumin in patients with advanced pancreatic cancer." *Clinical Cancer Research* 14.14 (2008): 4491-4499.

14. Sandur, Santosh K., et al. "Curcumin modulates the radiosensitivity of colorectal cancer cells by suppressing constitutive and inducible NF-κB activity." *International Journal of Radiation Oncology* Biology* Physics* 75.2 (2009): 534-542.

15. Kuderer, Nicole M., et al. "A meta-analysis and systematic review of the efficacy and safety of anticoagulants as cancer treatment." *Cancer* 110.5 (2007): 1149-1161.

16. Atiba, Ayman, et al. "Aloe vera oral administration accelerates acute radiation-delayed wound healing by stimulating transforming growth factor-β and fibroblast growth factor production." *The American Journal of Surgery* 201.6 (2011): 809-818.

17. Overgaard, Jens, et al. "Randomised trial of hyperthermia as adjuvant to radiotherapy for recurrent or metastatic malignant melanoma." *The Lancet* 345.8949 (1995): 540-543.

18. Overgaard, Jens. "Simultaneous and sequential hyperthermia and radiation treatment of an experimental tumor and its surrounding normal tissue in vivo." *International Journal of Radiation Oncology* Biology* Physics* 6.11 (1980): 1507-1517.

19. Hurwitz, Mark, and Paul Stauffer. "Hyperthermia, Radiation and Chemo-
    therapy: The Role of Heat in Multidisciplinary Cancer Care." *Seminars in
    oncology*. Vol. 41. No. 6. WB Saunders, 2014.

Chapter 6

Surgery Support

"Everything's physical manifestation reflects its inner essence."
- Jakob Bohme

I have had many cases in my practice where it was necessary to convince patients that surgery is the best option. If there is a localized cancerous mass that is easily accessible through surgery, then removing that mass is your best chance of a cure. One case that stands out was a young woman that came to my office with a pancreatic tumour that was unlikely to metastasize. She was trying a number of different natural therapies and the tumour was continuing to grow at a rapid rate. The mass was causing her significant pain and discomfort. She came to my office in tears from the pain and she was constantly nauseous with frequent vomiting. It was clear that at this point in time, her only option was surgery.

When I recommended the surgery she immediately began to cry and became defensive. She insisted that she did not want surgery. I wish that there were something natural that would be as effective as surgery in this case, but the reality is that this was her only option. For her this was unacceptable news and the last thing that she wanted to hear. It is not my job to tell the patient what they want to hear. It is my job to tell them what they need to hear. This was a clear example of a patient being told what they did not want to hear. Fortunately, I know that this conversation led to her eventual decision to get the surgery. I was happy to hear that she was able to overcome her resistance and get the treatment that she so desperately needed.

Surgery is sometimes necessary, and depending on the procedure, it can take quite some time for patients to heal. The best chance of a cure is almost always surgery. If there is an opportunity to remove the mass with good margins, then the patient should take advantage of this opportunity. Where surgery becomes controversial is when the data suggests that there is a possibility of metastasis. Unfortunately current diagnostic imaging is unable to guarantee that there are no metastatic sites. A mass of several million cells would be completely undetectable by any current diagnostic tool. As a result, we must base the decision on statistics and characteristics of the specific type of cancer. Some cancers are much more likely to spread than others. All of this must be factored in when considering surgery as an option.

Generally speaking, if there are multiple cancerous sites then surgery is not recommended. If surgery is unlikely to remove all cancerous cells, then the surgery is unlikely to be curative. There is evidence to suggest that the primary tumour releases chemical signals that inhibit the growth of smaller sites in the body. It is almost as if the main tumour is greedy and working hard to make sure that it gets all the resources, leaving none for the smaller tumours. When the main mass is removed, this often eliminates the inhibitory signal and the smaller masses suddenly start to grow at a more rapid rate. It is for this reason that surgery is rarely recommended if it is not possible to remove all the cells of concern. Of course there are exceptions to this rule and sometimes chemotherapy is beneficial after surgery. If the major mass is removed, then sometimes the chemotherapy can control these smaller masses and prevent them from advancing.

There is certainly a time and a place for surgery, but it is a major procedure and the decision to proceed should not be taken lightly. The patient needs to be able to whole-heartedly embrace the surgery as their cure. They should be ready mentally and physically for the procedure. If there is an opportunity to remove the entire mass, then the patient should take advantage of that opportunity as soon as possible. This means that physical and mental preparations should begin right away to make sure that every cell in the body is ready for the surgery.

It is important for every patient to know that there are therapies available which promote wound healing post surgery. Every surgical procedure is stressful on the body and this stress changes the metabolic requirements in your cells. As the body puts energy into wound healing, the demand for several nutrients suddenly increases. For optimal wound healing, it is essential that these nutrients are supplied.

Collagen is a key component of the wound healing process. Vitamin C is essential post surgery as it is required for proper collagen formation[1,2]. The enzymes that produce and stabilize collagen require significant amounts of Vitamin C. It is well established that patients who smoke are slower to heal from surgery. This is because cigarette smoke is oxidative which results in a rapid depletion of Vitamin C in the tissues[3]. With inadequate supplies of this essential nutrient, the collagen is slow to form and the collagen that does form tends to be weak. As a consequence, the wounds are more likely to break open after surgery due to their inability to effectively heal. It has been known for decades that when patients are supplemented with Vitamin C, they heal faster after surgery[4].

Another nutrient that is important with regards to wound healing is zinc. Many of the enzymes that are directly required for wound healing are dependent on a sufficient supply of zinc. Patients with a genetic predisposition to zinc deficiency have significantly impaired wound healing capabilities[5]. After a traumatic event such as surgery, the requirements for zinc in the body are significantly higher. When patients are supplemented with zinc they heal faster as they are able to meet this obvious metabolic requirement[5]. Not only is zinc helpful for wound healing, it is also effective at stimulating the immune system. It is essential that the immune system remain strong after a surgical procedure and the zinc will help maintain the strength of the immune cells.

Vitamin A is another nutrient that must be supplied in adequate amounts for proper wound healing to occur. Patients with a deficiency in Vitamin A are less efficient at healing wounds[6]. The role of Vitamin A in wound healing is different than that of zinc and Vitamin C. It is likely that the wound healing properties of Vitamin A are due to its ability to regulate the immune system locally in a way that is conducive to tissue repair.

Not only should patients be supplemented with these basic nutrients, their diet should be altered to help promote tissue healing as well. The patient must significantly increase their protein intake while avoiding inflammatory foods. It is not unusual for patients to struggle with protein consumption after a surgery. Eating can be uncomfortable and sometimes the appetite can be diminished as a result. In these circumstances, sometimes supplemental IV therapies can greatly aid in the healing process. By using only a couple of IV treatments, this can effectively ensure that the patient gets adequate levels of all the nutrients necessary to heal. A typical

IV solution would contain Vitamin C, zinc and a moderate amount of B-vitamins to help facilitate the wound healing process.

All of these simple changes make a profound difference in the healing process. These natural approaches are well supported by scientific evidence but they are not commonly encouraged by surgeons. This is often due to their lack of training in nutrition. If you have an upcoming surgery make sure that you contact a Naturopathic doctor to help you develop a plan that will accelerate your healing after the surgery is complete. It is critical to have professional guidance when you are preparing for a surgery. The dose and the quality of the supplements make a huge difference. Some of the recommended approaches are contraindicated in certain conditions, and it takes an expert to develop a plan that is both safe and effective for you.

Intravenous Nutrient Support

There are some circumstances where patients have disturbances in the gastrointestinal tract which make it difficult for them to absorb nutrients. The requirement for nutrients is very high for wound healing so it is imperative that patients get these nutrients into their cells. Sometimes the best way to do this is to bypass the digestive tract all together by putting these nutrients directly into the veins.

After any abdominal surgery, the digestive tract will not be able to digest and absorb nutrients efficiently. The significant inflammation that occurs as a result of surgery will impair the absorption of many critical nutrients. It is also important to point out that often after a surgery, it is not unusual for patients to have a diminished or altered appetite. Sometimes they will simply lose interest in the foods that they desperately need. Often they will still heal from the surgery but by supplying the appropriate nutrients, it is possible to speed up the healing process significantly.

By putting all of the essential nutrients into an intravenous infusion the patient gets these nutrients directly into their blood stream. Even for patients with no health concerns in the digestive tract, it can still be helpful to give some extra vitamins and nutrients through the veins. These are not mega doses, but they are sufficient to saturate the cells with the necessary nutrients.

Before surgery there are a couple of unique safety concerns that must be considered. It is critical to make sure that no supplements or intravenous therapies are going to interfere with the anesthetics. The reality is at normal therapeutic doses these concerns are minimal but you must have a Naturopathic physician go through all the supplements that you are on to make sure that there are no interactions. At very high doses of IV Vitamin C there are concerns that this could increase the risk of bleeding. A more thorough review of the evidence downplays the significance of this interaction; however, it is still helpful to be aware of this. The doses of IV Vitamin C required for surgery preparation are not high enough to be of concern. The few grams of Vitamin C in the IV infusion will significantly help with healing after the surgery and it carries minimal risk. The reason that IV therapies are so effective is that the nutrients are being directly infused into the blood stream.

Modified Citrus Pectin before Cancer Surgery

During any surgery there is always a risk of complications and with cancer surgery, there is also a risk of spreading the disease. The good news is that there are supplements that can help to reduce the risk of metastasis. Perhaps the most critical supplement to reduce the risk of metastasis is modified citrus pectin (MCP)[9]. This is a supplement that is not commonly recommended by surgeons, but the evidence for its efficacy is overwhelming.

The mechanism of MCP is well understood and it is a potent inhibitor of Galectin-3[16]. This is an adhesion molecule that is greatly over expressed on the surface of cancerous cells. Not only does MCP reduce the risk of metastasis, but it also slows down the rate of growth of metastatic cancer. If any cancerous cell is dislodged, then it needs to attach to a tissue where it can establish a blood supply before it grows into a tumour. The MCP helps to inhibit the actual attachment of the cancerous cell to tissues distant from the tumour site. Not only is the use of this supplement helpful in preparation for surgery, it can also slow down the rate of cancerous spread even in advanced cases[7,8].

Every cell has molecules on its surface that are specifically designed to adhere to other cells or to the extra cellular environment. The MCP is loaded with molecules called pectins which interact with these surface receptors. By adhering to these adhesion molecules on the surface of cells, the MCP makes the cells less sticky. This makes it less likely for a cancerous cell to establish a metastasis at a distant site. A good analogy to this concept is simple scotch tape. When the tape is clean it is sticky and it will stick to virtually any surface. If someone were to sprinkle some dust on that same piece of tape, then it would not be sticky at all. This is exactly what you are doing to your cells when you take modified citrus pectin.

Ultimately the goal of integrative cancer care is to support the patient through the surgery. We want to look at all the different factors in that patient's life and see how we can modify every factor to promote the healing process and reduce the risk of complications. Adding MCP into the protocol can help to reduce the possibility of complications, and the surgery preparation protocol will help to promote wound healing from the surgery itself. There are few professional grade products of MCP that are of sufficient quality. It is critical that you have professional guidance when choosing an MCP product.

Recently I heard an interesting story from a colleague who prescribed MCP to a patient in preparation for surgery. This was a palliative surgery as the cancer had already spread to many sites throughout the body. This patient misunderstood the directions from his doctor and continued to take MCP for years. Amazingly he remained stable for years even in this advanced stage. After several years, he decided to discontinue the supplement, and shortly after, the cancer rapidly progressed and he passed away. Although this is not how MCP is typically prescribed, it is helpful to note that it has applications beyond surgery. It can be an effective tool to slow down the progression of metastatic cancers in some cases.

Gotu Kola and Wounds

Gotu Kola, also known as Centella asiatica, grows in tropical swampy areas in Southeast Asia. It is an ancient remedy that has been used for centuries to help heal wounds. There is an abundance of scientific literature which supports the fact that Gotu Kola significantly speeds up the rate of healing[10,11].

The exact mechanism for this healing effect is poorly understood, but the overall effect is well documented. It appears that a subset of molecules in Gotu Kola called triterpenes significantly stimulate extracellular matrix accumulation in wounds[12]. This is one of the first steps that is necessary for a wound to heal. Shortly after experiencing a wound, the body will recruit cells called fibroblasts to the area in an effort to heal that wound. These same triterpenes from Gotu Kola have also demonstrated that they can stimulate fibroblasts to produce more collagen[13].

Another effect from this ancient remedy is that it can help with cognition. The mechanism of this improved cognition is unclear but it is thought to be related to the antioxidant effects of this herb[14]. This property is certainly relevant to surgery, because after a major procedure, it is not unusual for patients to have impaired cognition while the body focuses on healing.

This herb can be applied topically or it can be taken orally and both methods appear to have significant benefits. The best route of administering this should be determined by your Naturopathic doctor. Gotu Kola is metabolized through the liver and as a result there is potential for interaction with prescription medications. When used appropriately, it is a safe remedy that can help increase the rate of healing. There are several properties about the wound that must be considered before determining the most appropriate method of administration.

Aloe Vera and Scars

Many patients become self-conscious about the scars that result from a surgery. It is important to be patient because it takes a long time for the body to fully heal. After a surgery the wound healing process can take over two years to complete. The first three days consist of the hemostasis phase where essentially the body focuses its efforts on stopping the bleeding. The next 20 days are known as the inflammation phase, where a new framework is established for blood vessel growth. From week one to week six the wound starts to close with scar tissue and this is known as the proliferation phase of wound healing. The final stage of wound healing is known as the remodeling phase, which starts on week six and continues for the next two years.

Initially this timeline seems unreasonably long, but stop and think about it for a second. It does not take a surgeon to recognize the difference between a recent scar and an old scar. The recent scars appear red or raised and the old scars are flat and pale in colour. This transition to an old scar takes a very long time as the body remodels the scar tissue to be more consistent with the surrounding tissue.

The good news is that there are a number of natural therapies that can help to minimize the appearance of such scars. Application of aloe vera to a scar can help to promote the wound healing process while reducing the inflammation associated with the scar[15]. In my experience, the most noticeable change resulting from the application of aloe is that the scar loses its reddened colour. It tends to accelerate the transition from a red raised scar to a flattened lighter scar.

Scar tissue unfortunately will never be as strong as the surrounding tissue. No matter how many supplements are used or time given to heal, a scar will never be as strong. Healthy tissue has a coordinated arrangement of connective tissue that maintains the tissue integrity. Scar tissue consists of collagen and fibrinogen that is rapidly deposited to heal the wound. This uncoordinated arrangement will never be able to reach the same tissue strength as before the wound. This is why we must work hard to support the wound healing process so that the scar tissue can become as strong as possible.

Just like Gotu Kola, aloe vera can be taken orally or applied topically. Both methods have demonstrated a consistent positive effect on wound healing from surgeries. Many patients find the gel directly from the aloe plant to be more effective than aloe creams. If you have access to an aloe plant, I would certainly recommend using the gel directly from the plant. Aloe can also be helpful to promote healing of radiation burns, but remember this can only be applied after the radiation is complete. It is very dangerous to apply any oil to the skin prior to radiation and you will not be able to adequately wash it all off. This is something that every patient undergoing radiation should be aware of!

Another technique that can be used to improve the appearance of scars is neural therapy. This is a technique that involves injecting the scar tissue with procaine (a local anesthetic). By injecting this fluid directly into the scar tissue, it breaks up the scar tissue and it gives the collagen another chance to align more effectively. I have personally witnessed some dramatic improvements in patients who have used this technique. However, it is important not to use neural therapy until the wound is sufficiently healed.

The human body is not designed to go through such an intense procedure as surgery. Where in nature would we sustain such a significant injury and survive? It simply would not happen. As a result, we need to assist the body in this healing process using every tool at our disposal.

Post Surgery Complications

Many patients are left completely unaware of how long the effects from surgery will persist after the procedure. The actual scar tissue will be remodeling for up to two years after surgery. To the patient this will feel like nothing is changing because they are dealing with the aftermath of surgery on a daily basis. However, if you carefully document changes, you will often notice a slow and steady improvement over the course of two years.

A common example of this delayed healing time is with a surgery known as a proctectomy. This is when the entire prostate is removed in patients with prostate cancer. Surgeons will often describe to patients that they will do the "nerve sparing" procedure and people assume that this means the nerves will be unharmed, so that an erection is still possible. A nerve sparing procedure simply means that they will not sever the nerve. They focus a significant effort on maintaining the health of the nerves, but these delicate nerves are often damaged by the procedure even though they were not directly cut.

After a nerve sparing proctectomy it is not unusual for patients to have erectile dysfunction that persists for more than four years after the procedure. It takes a long time for the scar tissue and nerves to heal and it is important to be patient with the healing process. All of these natural therapies can help to facilitate the healing process and reduce the risk of complications, but the body still needs time to heal from such an invasive procedure as surgery.

Summary:

- Vitamin C is often the rate limiting step in the formation of scar tissue and it is essential that the body is adequately supplied with this nutrient before and after surgery
- Vitamin A helps to speed up the rate of healing by regulating the immune system in the local region of the scar
- Zinc must be supplied to cells to help with the formation of scar tissue and to support the immune system
- Modified citrus pectin used prior to surgery helps reduce the risk of metastasis
- If absorption of nutrients is an issue, then it may be necessary to get these vitamins and nutrients through intravenous administration
- Aloe vera and Gotu Kola helps heal scars when taken either orally or applied topically
- The wound healing process continues for over two years after surgery

References:

1. MacKay, Douglas, and Alan L. Miller. "Nutritional support for wound healing." Alternative medicine review: a *journal of clinical therapeutic* 8.4 (2003): 359-377.

2. Boyera, N., I. Galey, and B. A. Bernard. "Effect of vitamin C and its derivatives on collagen synthesis and cross-linking by normal human fibroblasts." *International Journal of Cosmetic Science* 20.3 (1998): 151-158.

3. Schectman, Gordon, James C. Byrd, and Harvey W. Gruchow. "The influence of smoking on vitamin C status in adults." *American Journal of Public Health* 79.2 (1989): 158-162.

4. Bartlett, Marshall K., Chester M. Jones, and Anna E. Ryan. "Vitamin C and wound healing: II. Ascorbic acid content and tensile strength of healing wounds in human beings." *New England Journal of Medicine* 226.12 (1942): 474-481.

5. Lansdown, Alan BG, et al. "Zinc in wound healing: theoretical, experimental, and clinical aspects." *Wound Repair and Regeneration* 15.1 (2007): 2-16.

6. Hunt, Thomas K. "Vitamin A and wound healing." *Journal of the American Academy of Dermatology* 15.4 (1986): 817-821.

7. Nangia-Makker, Pratima, et al. "Inhibition of human cancer cell growth and metastasis in nude mice by oral intake of modified citrus pectin." *Journal of the National Cancer Institute* 94.24 (2002): 1854-1862.

8. Azémar, Marc, et al. "Clinical benefit in patients with advanced solid tumors treated with modified citrus pectin: a prospective pilot study." *Clin Med: Oncol* 1 (2007): 73-80.

9. Kidd, P. "A new approach to metastatic cancer prevention: modified citrus pectin (MCP), a unique pectin that blocks cell surface lectins." *Altern Med* Rev 1 (1996): 4-10.

10. Suguna, L., P. Sivakumar, and G. Chandrakasan. "Effects of Centella asiatica extract on dermal wound healing in rats." *Indian Journal of Experimental Biology* 34.12 (1996): 1208-1211.

11. Shukla, A., et al. "In vitro and in vivo wound healing activity of asiaticoside isolated from Centella asiatica." *Journal of ethnopharmacology* 65.1 (1999): 1-11.

12. Maquart, F. X., et al. "Triterpenes from Centella asiatica stimulate extracellular matrix accumulation in rat experimental wounds." *European Journal of Dermatology* 9.4 (1999): 289-96.

13. Maquart, Francois-Xavier, et al. "Stimulation of collagen synthesis in fibroblast cultures by a triterpene extracted from Centella asiatica." *Connective tissue research* 24.2 (1990): 107-120.

14. Kumar, MH Veerendra, and Y. K. Gupta. "Effect of different extracts of Centella asiatica on cognition and markers of oxidative stress in rats." *Journal of Ethnopharmacology* 79.2 (2002): 253-260.

15. Davis, Robert H., et al. "Anti-inflammatory and wound healing activity of a growth substance in Aloe vera." *Journal of the American Podiatric Medical Association* 84 (1994): 77-81.

16. Hossein, Ghamartaj, et al. "Synergistic effects of PectaSol-C modified citrus pectin an inhibitor of Galectin-3 and paclitaxel on apoptosis of human SKOV-3 ovarian cancer cells." *Asian Pac J Cancer* Prev 14.12 (2013): 7561-8.

Surgery Support

Chapter 7

Prescription Medications and Cancer

**"Our task is not to treat the disease,
but the patient."**
- Vincent Preissnitz

When used appropriately there are several prescription medications that are helpful as adjunctive cancer therapies. Many of them help to reduce the side effects of chemotherapy while increasing its effectiveness. I have a patient who is on a long-term maintenance dose of chemotherapy. When I first saw her she was against taking any prescription medication. I found it curious that she was so quick to take chemotherapy, yet so adamantly against taking a gentle prescription given for heartburn. She initially feared the side effects from a heartburn medication more than the side effects from the chemotherapy. I presented her with research about how useful this drug can be in her specific case but she continued to refuse over a long period of time.

When she reached her sixteenth cycle, she started to get really worn down from all the side effects of chemotherapy. It was not until these side effects became unbearable that she decided to take my advice. Once she started this simple adjunctive therapy, she almost immediately noticed the difference, making it much easier for her to continue with the chemotherapy. In all of her cycles since, she has been almost symptom free and is no longer fearful of continuing the maintenance chemotherapy. When the right adjunctive therapy is used, patients often notice a positive change rather quickly. This helps to make the conventional treatments more tolerable and more effective.

There are several different prescription medications that have compelling research to support their use as an adjunctive cancer therapy. These uses would be considered off label but the mechanism of action makes sense on a biochemical level. There is an abundance of research to support the use of these medications and it is interesting to see how they are used differently around the world.

In North America, it seems that many of these adjunctive cancer therapies are rarely used but this is not the case in other parts of the world. For example, in Asia it is the standard of care to use the heartburn medication cimetidine in conjunction with the chemotherapy 5-FU. In Europe, it is common for oncologists to use the COX-2 inhibitor Celebrex with platinum chemotherapies. These are just a few examples of prescription medications that have applications as an adjunctive cancer therapy. It is important to point out that every one of these medications has potential interactions, and it takes an experienced Naturopathic physician to know if these medications are appropriate for you.

Diabetes Medications and Cancer

Can drugs traditionally used for diabetes also be helpful with cancer? There is a growing body of evidence which indicates that both metformin and a class of drugs known as thiazolidinediones can be a useful adjunctive cancer therapy. The biochemical mechanism behind this anti-cancer effect is poorly defined but there are some intriguing theories about the mechanism of action.

Metformin is the first line drug for patients with type 2 diabetes and it is certainly effective at regulating blood sugar levels. Diabetic patients who regularly take metformin have a lower risk of developing cancer[1]. Metformin activates an enzyme known as AMPK. A recent breakthrough has found a key regulator of AMPK to be a protein known as LKB1. LKB1 is a well-recognized tumour suppressor. Activation of AMPK by metformin and exercise requires LKB1, and this would also explain why exercise is beneficial in the primary and secondary prevention of certain cancers[2]. In other words, metformin activates some of the same molecular pathways which become active during exercise. Although metformin is not a replacement for exercise, by stimulating these same pathways this can explain some of the positive benefits of metformin in the context of cancer.

Recent studies strongly indicate that the anti-cancer effects of metformin are indeed linked to AMPK[3]. Metformin appears to selectively target cancer stem cells and acts together with chemotherapy to block tumour growth and prolong remission[4]. When used with doxorubicin, it acts synergistically to reduce tumour mass and reduce relapse rates. This synergy is more effective than either drug alone. Metformin is often used as an adjunctive cancer therapy in breast cancer patients who have adequate kidney function.

Metformin is generally well tolerated, and there is no risk of causing hypoglycemia. It has a long history of safe use and the most common side effect is gas and bloating. In patients who cannot tolerate these symptoms, there is another form of this drug called Glumetza. This is a slow release version of metformin and it gradually releases the medication rather than rapidly delivering it all at once. Glumetza is often well tolerated by patients who did not tolerate standard metformin medication.

There is a completely different class of medications used for diabetes that also has anti-cancer effects. The drug class is known as thiazolidinediones. One of the most well known drugs in this class is called Avandia. There has been some recent controversy about this drug due an increase in cardiovascular events after prolonged use. Even though metformin and Avandia are effective at treating diabetes they work by completely different mechanisms. The thiazolidinediones activate a receptor called PPAR which triggers a cascade of reactions that are beneficial to patients fighting cancer[6,7,8]. The drug increases the activity of a key tumour suppressor called PTEN[5]. This tumour suppressor is a protein that halts the growth of cancer cells by inhibiting an enzyme known as PI3K. There are many types of cancer that are dependent on inhibiting the function of the tumour suppressor PTEN. The bottom line is that this drug helps to put the brakes on the growth of cancerous cells by activating PTEN.

As more research accumulates supporting the fact that these anti-diabetic drugs can be used to treat cancer, one thing is becoming clear: The anti-cancer effect from these drugs is due to their influence on several different metabolic pathways. The great thing about these medications is that they have a long history of use and they are well established as safe adjunctive cancer therapies. Like any medication, it has to be used in the right context and these therapies are not for everyone. These medications should not be used prior to a PET scan because it can alter the metabolism of sugar in the body. Normally this change in metabolism of sugar is a positive change, but it can alter the results of these scans. If metformin is discontinued 48 hours before the scan, then it will not affect the results because it has a short half-life in the body. It is necessary to have a Naturopathic doctor go through your entire case history to determine if these treatments are indicated for you.

Low Dose Naltrexone

Naltrexone is typically used for patients with opioid or alcohol dependence. It is a molecule that powerfully counteracts the effects of opioids. At lower doses this drug can be used with cancer patients to help balance the immune system and inhibit the growth of cancer[9]. There are many well documented cases in the scientific literature of patients surviving years longer than expected after using low dose naltrexone (LDN)[10,12]. This therapy is rapidly becoming mainstream as more research accumulates supporting its use in cancer.

The mechanism of the anti-cancer effect of LDN is not completely understood. It is thought that the LDN targets the opioid growth factor receptor pathway to inhibit cell proliferation in cancerous cells[13]. There is also evidence to suggest that at these lower doses the immune system is modulated in a way that is beneficial to fighting cancer[11]. These positive changes in the immune system from LDN have also been shown to make a positive difference in patients with Multiple Sclerosis and HIV. The bottom line is that when used appropriately, it can be an effective therapy in an integrative cancer setting.

When LDN is used in conjunction with alpha lipoic acid (ALA) it can be a potent therapy for pancreatic cancer. There are a number of case studies where patients with metastatic pancreatic cancer have survived many years longer than expected using only this therapy[10,12]. LDN is commonly used for lymphoma when patients are not on opioids for pain management. There are also several studies that support the use of LDN with ovarian cancer, and preliminary research indicates that it works synergistically with the chemotherapy cisplatin[9].

The side effects from naltrexone are minimal when taken at low doses. Often cancer patients will take 3mg before bed and sometimes this results in vivid dreams. The most common side effect is loose stools which is not surprising given the mechanism of the drug. Opioid medications often cause extreme constipation due to stimulation of the opioid receptors. Low dose naltrexone does the opposite by inhibiting the opioid receptors and loose stools can be a consequence of this. A significant number of cancer patients tend to be constipated due to the medications and, as a result, the "laxative effect" of the LDN is usually not a serious concern.

It is important to recognize that this therapy is not for everyone. Many cancer patients are treated with opioids for pain management. Given that this drug acts as an opioid antagonist, it is not indicated for patients on opioid medication such as morphine. It would directly counteract the effects of this important pain medication. When LDN is used in the appropriate cellular context, it can be an effective adjunctive cancer therapy.

Heartburn and Cancer

Many cancer patients undergoing chemotherapy have constant disturbances in their gastrointestinal tract. Heartburn is common in these patients and it is frequently treated with a class of drugs called proton pump inhibitors (PPI's). Some common PPI's are Pariet, Losec, Nexium and Tecta. There is no question that these drugs are effective at controlling heartburn symptoms. These drugs dramatically suppress the stomach's ability to produce acid. When patients are on these drugs long-term, it can be difficult to discontinue them because heartburn symptoms reappear whenever they miss a dose. In the context of cancer, there are other options that can be considered before using PPI's.

There is a class of drugs called H2-receptor antagonists and these drugs are also effective at reducing stomach acid production. The reduction in stomach acid tends to be short term and patients do not become as dependent on these medications as compared to PPI's. The most researched heartburn medication in the context of cancer is cimetidine, also known as Tagamet. There is a substantial body of evidence which indicates that Tagamet is an effective adjunctive cancer therapy[19,20,21,22]. The conclusion from one major study was [19]:

> These results clearly indicate that cimetidine treatment dramatically improved survival in colorectal cancer patients with tumour cells expressing high levels of sLx and sLa. (Matsumoto 161)

An interesting double blind study was completed in 1988 which showed that survival was significantly enhanced in patients who took cimetidine for two years after gastric cancer surgery[24]. Many of these gastrointestinal cancers are stimulated by histamine, and cimetidine blocks this effect[25]. The use of cimetidine as an adjunctive cancer therapy is often indicated for gastric and colon cancers.

Cimetidine is thought to target a class of molecules known as cadherins and by doing so it reduces the risk of metastasis. In Asia, cimetidine is used in conjunction with the chemotherapy 5-FU to treat colorectal cancers and this has resulted in significant improvements in patient survival[19]. It appears that there are several other pathways involved with this anti-cancer effect. Regardless of the mechanism, it is clear that this medication has potential as an adjunctive cancer therapy in patients with colorectal cancer.

Cimetidine is not appropriate for everyone as there are a number of potential interactions. It is metabolized through the P450 pathways[23] and these are the same pathways that many other drugs are metabolized through. This is not an absolute contraindication but you should be careful about the dosing. It is often best to slowly introduce cimetidine. It is essential that you have a Naturopathic physician who is familiar with the use of cimetidine to review your medications and determine if this is the right therapy for you.

Controlling Tumour Inflammation with Celebrex

Tumours often have a significant amount of inflammation surrounding these abnormal cells. This inflammation can make the tumour seem larger than it is and cause significant complications if it starts to impinge on nerves or blood vessels. This inflammation allows the cancer to be more invasive, making it easier for the cancerous cells to evade the immune system. Oncologists around the world are working hard to address the inflammation that is associated with cancer. There are already several prescription medications that are showing some encouraging results when it comes to addressing the cancer inflammation problem. One of those prescriptions is celecoxib, also known as Celebrex.

Celebrex is a selective COX-2 non-steroidal anti-inflammatory (NSAID). It is commonly used to treat joint pain and more recently research has shown that it has potential as an adjunctive cancer therapy. Initially this drug was developed with the intention of being a safer NSAID. Commonly used NSAIDs such as ibuprofren and Aspirin will significantly increase the risk of severe gastrointestinal bleeding. It was thought that the risk of gastrointestinal bleeding was due to the fact that these NSAIDs influence COX-1 and COX-2. The logic was that if a drug was developed to be selective for COX-2 then the risk of bleeding would decrease.

It turns out that they were incorrect about this assumption. Not only does the COX-2 specific drug Celebrex have an increased risk of gastrointestinal bleeds (just like its non-selective predecessors) it also increases the risk of cardiovascular events. Recently Celebrex has received a lot of negative press about the increased risks that come with long-term use. In the context of general health, it is probably best to find an alternative to Celebrex if you intend to use it long-term. However, when someone is faced with a serious diagnosis of cancer and they intend to only use the drug for a short period of time, then the benefits certainly outweigh the risks.

The mechanism behind this anti-cancer effect appears to be due to several different metabolic pathways. The most prominent pathway is its inhibition of AKT signalling which induces apoptosis and enhances the effectiveness of several chemotherapies including paclitaxel and carboplatin[26,27,28]. The inflammation surrounding tumours helps to facilitate metastasis of cancerous cells. Celebrex appears to help reduce the invasiveness of tumours by controlling the inflammation in the tumour microenvironment. Inflammation in the microenvironment of a tumour is so ubiquitous that some are even calling for cancer related inflammation to be considered a hallmark of cancer[29].

Although this drug can be used as an adjunctive cancer therapy in gastrointestinal cancers, it is not safe for everyone. It is contraindicated in patients with allergies to sulfonamides and patients with active gastrointestinal bleeds. There are a handful drug interactions with Celebrex because it is metabolized by the same metabolic pathway as many other common medications. This is certainly not an absolute contraindication and if it is gradually introduced while the patient is monitored, then it can be used safely. These interactions are worth mentioning; however, it is important to consider that in a typical poly-pharmacy cancer case, the interactions with Celebrex are often minor compared to the interactions between various chemotherapies and pain medications.

The Dangers of DHEA

DHEA is often described as a wonder drug that is used by patients interested in its anti-aging effects. As we age, the levels of DHEA in the blood start to decrease. The logic was that if patients were given this hormone, they would be able to partially reverse the aging process. There is evidence to suggest that indeed it does improve many of the characteristics that we associate with aging.

Supplementation with DHEA is not safe for everyone as it is strongly associated with an increased risk of developing breast cancer[14,15]. In response to this risk, supplement companies began to produce a molecule called 7-keto DHEA, which is a metabolite of DHEA. This was considered a safer alternative to DHEA because it does not break down into estrogen or testosterone[17]. It is true that when patients take 7-keto DHEA, there is no statistically significant increase in hormone levels, but this does not make it safe to use for breast cancer patients (or any other hormone dependent cancer).

I have personally seen several patients with active estrogen positive breast cancer who were prescribed 7-keto DHEA by a Medical doctor. This is a dangerous combination and it is reckless to prescribe this medication in this clinical situation. 7-keto DHEA is not safe for any patient with estrogen positive breast cancer. There are a number of obvious biochemical reasons for this contraindication. First of all there are absolutely no studies which indicate that this is safe with estrogen positive breast cancer. Secondly, just because the estrogen levels are not elevated does not mean that the estrogen receptors are not being stimulated.

Normally the receptors on the surface of a cell are only stimulated by a few specific molecules. The estrogen receptors are notoriously promiscuous. What this means is that they are stimulated by many different molecules other than estrogen. One of those molecules is 7-keto DHEA. In other words, even though patients do not have elevations in their estrogen levels, the estrogen receptors are being directly stimulated by the 7-keto DHEA[16]. As far as the cancer cells are concerned, they will act as if they are being stimulated by estrogen even though the actual levels of estrogen remain unchanged.

In one study it was conclusively shown that 7-keto DHEA (aka 7-oxo DHEA) is a low affinity ligand activator of estrogen receptors. The estrogen activity in these cancer cell lines was significantly elevated compared to the controls. In this same study, the cancer cells (MCF-7 breast cancer cells) that were treated with 7-keto DHEA grew much faster than the controls. This study certainly raises concerns about the use of this supplement in cancer patients. It is clearly misleading to state that 7-keto DHEA has all the positive effects of DHEA without any of the negative effects. This is simply not how our cells operate on the biochemical level.

Another obvious concern is that 7-keto DHEA is essentially structurally identical to DHEA. This means that its overall molecular shape is so similar that it will stimulate estrogen receptors the same as if it was DHEA. The estrogen receptors on cancer cells cannot tell the difference between 7-keto DHEA and DHEA. As far as the cancer is concerned, it is the same thing. Of course the DHEA will not stimulate these receptors as strongly as estrogen, but they still increase the activity. This is the complete opposite of what you want to do with estrogen positive breast cancer. Conventional cancer therapies work very hard to reduce estrogen activity as much as possible because this acts as a signal for these cancer cells to grow[18].

It is important that more patients become aware of this serious concern, because it is difficult to sift through the mountains of information on the internet. Unfortunately, there are still doctors that are prescribing this medication to patients with hormone dependent cancers. The simple explanation that estrogen levels are unaffected does not mean that it is safe. Biology is much more complex than simply monitoring the level of a few arbitrary hormones in the blood. There is significant cross talk between these different metabolic pathways. This well understood biological concept also applies in a clinical setting. As a molecular biologist, I can tell you that these interactions are well documented and there is realistically no debate about this concept in the mainstream scientific community.

Summary:

- Metformin can be an effective adjunctive cancer therapy, especially in cases of breast cancer. It can work synergistically with the chemotherapy doxorubicin

- Avandia can be an adjunctive cancer therapy due to its activation of the tumour suppressor PTEN

- Low dose naltrexone can stimulate the immune system and it is particularly useful in cases of pancreatic cancer when combined with IV ALA

- Cimetidine is a heartburn medication that is synergistic with the chemotherapy 5-FU, especially in cases of colorectal cancer

- Celebrex is a selective COX-2 NSAID that reduces inflammation around tumours and it is synergistic with the chemotherapies paclitaxel and carboplatin

- DHEA should be strictly avoided in any hormone dependent cancer

References:

1. Evans, Josie MM, et al. "Metformin and reduced risk of cancer in diabetic patients." Bmj 330.7503 (2005): 1304-1305.

2. Bauman, Adrian E. "Updating the evidence that physical activity is good for health: an epidemiological review 2000–2003." *Journal of Science and Medicine in Sport* 7.1 (2004): 6-19.

3. Zakikhani, Mahvash, et al. "Metformin is an AMP kinase–dependent growth inhibitor for breast cancer cells." *Cancer research* 66.21 (2006): 10269-10273.

4. Hirsch, Heather A., et al. "Metformin selectively targets cancer stem cells, and acts together with chemotherapy to block tumor growth and prolong remission." *Cancer research* 69.19 (2009): 7507-7511.

5. Farrow, Buckminster, and B. Mark Evers. "Activation of PPARγ increases PTEN expression in pancreatic cancer cells." *Biochemical and biophysical research communications* 301.1 (2003): 50-53.

6. Bunt, Stephanie K., et al. "Rosiglitazone and Gemcitabine in combination reduces immune suppression and modulates T cell populations in pancreatic cancer." *Cancer Immunology, Immunotherapy* 62.2 (2013): 225-236.

7. Monami, Matteo, Ilaria Dicembrini, and Edoardo Mannucci. "Thiazolidinediones and cancer: results of a meta-analysis of randomized clinical trials." *Acta diabetologica* 51.1 (2014): 91-101.

8. Srivastava, Nishi, et al. "Inhibition of Cancer Cell Proliferation by PPARγ Is Mediated by a Metabolic Switch that Increases Reactive Oxygen Species Levels." *Cell metabolism* (2014).

9. Donahue, Renee N., Patricia J. McLaughlin, and Ian S. Zagon. "Low-dose naltrexone suppresses ovarian cancer and exhibits enhanced inhibition in combination with cisplatin." *Experimental Biology and Medicine* 236.7 (2011): 883-895.

10. Berkson, Burton M., Daniel M. Rubin, and Arthur J. Berkson. "The long-term survival of a patient with pancreatic cancer with metastases to the liver after treatment with the intravenous α-lipoic acid/low-dose naltrexone protocol." *Integrative cancer therapies* 5.1 (2006): 83-89.

11. Brown, Norman, and Jaak Panksepp. "Low-dose naltrexone for disease prevention and quality of life." *Medical hypotheses* 72.3 (2009): 333-337.

12. Berkson, Burton M., Daniel M. Rubin, and Arthur J. Berkson. "Revisiting the ALA/N (α-Lipoic Acid/Low-Dose Naltrexone) protocol for people with metastatic and nonmetastatic pancreatic cancer: a report of 3 new cases." *Integrative cancer therapies* 8.4 (2009): 416-422.

13. Donahue, Renee N., Patricia J. McLaughlin, and Ian S. Zagon. "Low-dose naltrexone targets the opioid growth factor–opioid growth factor receptor pathway to inhibit cell proliferation: mechanistic evidence from a tissue culture model." *Experimental Biology and Medicine* 236.9 (2011): 1036-1050.

14. Tworoger, Shelley S., et al. "The association of plasma DHEA and DHEA sulfate with breast cancer risk in predominantly premenopausal women." *Cancer Epidemiology Biomarkers & Prevention* 15.5 (2006): 967-971.

15. Key, T., et al. "Endogenous sex hormones and breast cancer in postmenopausal women: reanalysis of nine prospective studies." *Journal of the National Cancer Institute* 94.8 (2002): 606-616.

16. Michael Miller, Kristy K., et al. "DHEA metabolites activate estrogen receptors alpha and beta." *Steroids* 78.1 (2013): 15-25.

17. Lardy, Henry, et al. "Ergosteroids II: biologically active metabolites and synthetic derivatives of dehydroepiandrosterone." *Steroids* 63.3 (1998): 158-165.

18. Janni W, Hepp P. Adjuvant aromatase inhibitor therapy: Outcomes and safety. *Cancer Treat Rev.* 2010; 36:249–261.

19. Matsumoto, S., et al. "Cimetidine increases survival of colorectal cancer patients with high levels of sialyl Lewis-X and sialyl Lewis-A epitope expression on tumour cells." *British journal of cancer* 86.2 (2002): 161-167.

20. Kobayashi, Ken-ichi, et al. "Cimetidine inhibits cancer cell adhesion to endothelial cells and prevents metastasis by blocking E-selectin expression." *Cancer research* 60.14 (2000): 3978-3984.

21. Kubecova, Martina, et al. "Cimetidine: An anticancer drug?." European *Journal of Pharmaceutical Sciences* 42.5 (2011): 439-444.

22. Bolton, Elaine, Julie King, and David L. Morris. "H2-antagonists in the treatment of colon and breast cancer." *Seminars in cancer biology*. Vol. 10. No. 1. Academic Press, 2000.

23. Levine, Marc, et al. "In vivo cimetidine inhibits hepatic CYP2C6 and CYP2C11 but not CYP1A1 in adult male rats." *Journal of Pharmacology and Experimental Therapeutics* 284.2 (1998): 493-499.

24. Burtin, Claude, et al. "Clinical improvement in advanced cancer disease after treatment combining histamine and H2-antihistaminics (ranitidine or cimetidine)." *European Journal of Cancer and Clinical Oncology* 24.2 (1988): 161-167.

25. Adams, W. J., J. A. Lawson, and D. L. Morris. "Cimetidine inhibits in vivo growth of human colon cancer and reverses histamine stimulated in vitro and in vivo growth." *Gut* 35.11 (1994): 1632-1636.

26. Hsu, Ao-Lin, et al. "The cyclooxygenase-2 inhibitor celecoxib induces apoptosis by blocking Akt activation in human prostate cancer cells independently of Bcl-2." *Journal of Biological Chemistry* 275.15 (2000): 11397-11403.

27. Altorki, N. K., et al. "Celecoxib, a selective cyclo-oxygenase-2 inhibitor, enhances the response to preoperative paclitaxel and carboplatin in early-stage non–small-cell lung cancer." *Journal of clinical oncology* 21.14 (2003): 2645-2650.

28. Kulp, Samuel K., et al. "3-phosphoinositide-dependent protein kinase-1/Akt signaling represents a major cyclooxygenase-2-independent target for celecoxib in prostate cancer cells." *Cancer research* 64.4 (2004): 1444-1451.

29. Colotta, Francesco, et al. "Cancer-related inflammation, the seventh hallmark of cancer: links to genetic instability." *Carcinogenesis* 30.7 (2009): 1073-1081.

Chapter 8

Natural Supplements and Cancer

"We still do not know one thousandth of one percent of what nature has revealed to us."
- Albert Einstein

It was a cold January morning in Vancouver when I got a call from my grandmother. The roads were icy so my grandmother wanted me to give my grandfather a ride to the hospital for a doctor's appointment. I drove them to the appointment and afterwards I decided to stay over at their place for a cup of tea. At this point they were also happy to have company because they had been stranded in the apartment for several days due to unusually snowy weather. We began to talk about my grandfather's health. At 86 years old, he had congestive heart failure and the doctors were considering surgically implanting a pacemaker. Both of my grandparents are proactive about their health. On the kitchen counter there were over a dozen bottles of various supplements.

Being a student in Naturopathic medicine at the time, I had a solid understanding of these supplements and how they should be used. I went through all of their supplements and I was shocked at the low quality. Every supplement was an inexpensive brand and extremely low quality. These cheaper supplements are full of fillers which are molecules that serve no medicinal purpose. Some of the molecules were in a form that is poorly absorbed and in some cases harmful. One example was that their Vitamin E supplement only had alpha-tocopherol. This is only one of the eight different molecules that make up the Vitamin E complex.

A good Vitamin E supplement should contain mixed tocopherols and mixed tocotrienols, not just alpha-tocopherol. In fact, alpha-tocopherol supplementation has been associated with increased mortality rather than extending lifespan. If you ingest only alpha-tocopherol, it will displace the other fat soluble antioxidants, thus disrupting the antioxidant network. This will actually increase oxidative damage which is the complete opposite of what Vitamin E is supposed to do.

Scientists are eager to isolate the individual molecules that are responsible for the observed therapeutic benefits from any natural compound. Drug companies are always quick to jump on the bandwagon once a molecule is identified. The problem is that the optimal therapeutic benefit may not come from one molecule. As more molecules become identified and described, we are learning that it is the synergy of a complex network of molecules that is the most effective. Even in regard to Vitamin E, there are new factors just now being studied which show positive benefits. There are still many beneficial factors which have not even been discovered yet.

This got me thinking about clinical trials designed by those who are against nutraceuticals. Every once in a while you read a story in the mainstream media that says something like: "New study shows that this vitamin is ineffective or harmful...". In many of these negative trials, the researchers are using poor quality supplements. Some negative Vitamin E studies used supplements which contained only alpha-tocopherol.

One such study was labeled in the media as a negative study about the use of Vitamin E, but this is misleading. They were not actually studying Vitamin E because Vitamin E is a complex of molecules. They were studying one molecule called alpha-tocopherol. A good quality supplement uses mixed tocopherols and these higher quality studies are indeed showing positive benefits. It is not surprising that some clinical trials have disappointing results when they use low quality supplements.

My grandparents are intelligent and well educated people. In fact both of my grandparents are pharmacists and my grandfather finished at the top of his class. The problem is that neither pharmacists nor Medical doctors are properly educated on what a good supplement is. Often patients will hear that a supplement is good for their health, so they grab the first product that they see on the shelf at their local pharmacy.

Many doctors will read the headlines in the media of a poorly designed clinical trial which concluded that a supplement is useless or dangerous. As a result, they discourage all patients from taking it without having an understanding of the supplement or the details of the study. There is a lot of misinformation out there. If you browse the internet, you will easily find numerous articles written by uninformed individuals that express completely inaccurate and contradictory information.

This is why it is important to consult a health care professional who understands how to use high quality supplements which will make a positive difference in your life. Medical doctors simply do not receive adequate training in this important aspect of health. The employee at your local pharmacy or nutraceutical store will not have adequate knowledge in this area either. Not every supplement is appropriate for everyone, and it is essential that your treatment plan is customized to your unique set of conditions.

The supplements that I describe in this section are only a small subset of available treatments. There are many other supplements that have been demonstrated to be effective in an integrative oncology setting. These supplements are well supported by scientific evidence with a long history of safe and effective use. Please do not consult Dr. Google to develop your treatment plan. There is a lot of misleading and inaccurate information on the internet regarding cancer treatments. You need to contact a Naturopathic physician as they are knowledgeable in both medicine and supplements. A Naturopathic physician can guide you to high quality supplements that are right for you.

Micronutrient and Hormone Tests for Cancer

On a regular basis I have patients come into my office with the results from a micronutrient or hormone panel that was run by another physician. The results often show a seemingly random array of deficiencies. As a consequence, patients are often prescribed a number of supplements that are meant to fill in those nutritional gaps. This micronutrient approach may have some applications in the context of general health and well-being. However, I am skeptical about their use in the context of cancer.

There are several reasons why I do not recommend micronutrient and hormone panels for cancer patients. The first reason is that cancer is a complex disease and it will powerfully influence the biochemistry of every cell in the body. This major metabolic shift will almost certainly result in abnormal findings in a micronutrient or hormone test. These abnormal findings, however, do not mean that supplementation is indicated. These findings are simply an indication that the patient's overall metabolism is out of balance. Restoring this balance in a cancer patient is not as simple as replacing a perceived deficiency of a few hormones or nutrients.

If a cancer patient is deficient in a particular hormone or nutrient, this does not necessarily mean that he or she will benefit from supplementation of this nutrient. In fact, in many cases there is a reason for this deficiency. Low levels of certain nutrients could be your body's defence against the cancer. For example, cancer patients will often have low levels of iron. This does not mean that giving iron to these patients will help them! There is a time and a place to give iron and in some cases it is necessary to supplement patients with iron when they become too anemic.

The human body battles cancer by taking iron out of the blood. Low levels of iron in the blood represent a deliberate metabolic shift by your body to slow down the growth of cancer. Iron is needed for the initiation and the progression of cancer. Altered iron metabolism is one of the hallmark characteristics of cancer. In a patient fighting cancer, if you supplement with iron, then you are directly working against this natural defense mechanism.

Another common example of a metabolic shift during cancer is with DHEA levels. It is common for women with breast cancer to have low levels of DHEA. It is not unusual for these patients to also feel fatigued. This is not surprising considering the systemic inflammatory response that often occurs with cancer. Some physicians then mistakenly prescribe DHEA to help give the patient more energy and they justify it by the low levels of DHEA in the blood. The reason that the DHEA is low is because the cancer is shunting all the DHEA to make estrogen and promote growth of cancerous cells. This is another classic example of why low levels of a hormone or nutrient are not always an indication for supplementation. There is often a reason for these altered levels in the blood and in many cases we do not yet understand why the metabolism changes in these specific ways.

The bottom line is that these expensive tests do not provide any clinically useful information in the context of cancer. The results will not change the course of treatment, nor do they provide any information about the progression of the cancer. The levels will certainly be off, but this does not mean that it is necessary or helpful to bring these nutrients back to normal levels. Your treatment plan will be more effective if you are taking fewer supplements that are specifically indicated for your condition. When the body is fighting cancer, the absorption of nutrients is impaired and you can only absorb so many supplements to a therapeutic level. Your plan will be more effective if you are absorbing higher levels of supplements that we know will work, rather then supplying your body with small levels of minerals and nutrients based on an irrelevant test.

Quercetin

Quercetin is a bioflavonoid that is naturally found in a variety of fruits and vegetables. It has powerful effects on several specific biochemical pathways. Quercetin has potent antioxidant and anti-inflammatory properties. It has consistently been demonstrated to stimulate anti-tumour activities in the body.

Perhaps the most physiologically relevant target of quercetin is the transport protein p-glycoprotein. Every cell has a complex of proteins known as p-glycoproteins or multi-drug resistance protein 1 (MDR1) which actively pumps foreign substances out of cells. Cancer cells are toxic due to their irregular metabolism and as a result they have many of these transport molecules on their surface to remove toxins. The problem is that when cancer cells are treated with chemotherapy, the p-glycoprotein allows the cells to remove toxins before the drug has the opportunity to work. This simple mechanism allows cancer cells to survive in the presence of toxins and develop resistance to drugs.

Quercetin is a well documented inhibitor of p-glycoprotein[4,5]. In other words, when cancer cells are exposed to quercetin, they are no longer able to push the chemotherapy out as effectively. This results in an accumulation of chemotherapy within the cancer cells. When quercetin is combined with fasting and the appropriate chemotherapy, this can be a potent combination.

There is also evidence to suggest that quercetin slows down the rate of growth of rapidly dividing cells. Even at low doses, quercetin exerted cancer cell-specific inhibition of proliferation and this inhibition resulted from cell cycle arrest at the G1 phase[2]. The exact mechanism behind this effect is not fully understood, but it has been repeatedly observed in the scientific literature.

Quercetin also acts as an extremely potent heat shock protein inhibitor[6,7]. This is important because cancer cells are dependent on heat shock protein to survive in the warmer environment of the tumour. Normal cells are spatially arranged so that they can optimally displace heat. Tumour cells are densely packed together so they are inefficient at distributing heat. By inhibiting heat shock protein, quercetin can actually trigger cell death in cancerous cells. This supplement certainly has applications in hyperthermia treatment where cancer cells are significantly heated to make them more vulnerable to chemotherapy. This is discussed at length in the hyperthermia sections of chapters 4 (*Chemotherapy Support*) and 5 (*Radiation Support*).

Another useful effect of quercetin is that it acts as a natural aromatase inhibitor. After surgical removal of an estrogen positive breast cancer, it is common for women to be placed on an anti-estrogen therapy. The most commonly prescribed drugs are tamoxifen and letrozole. Tamoxifen works by blocking the estrogen receptor. Letrozole works by inhibiting an enzyme that produces estrogen. The net effect is that the activity of estrogen in the body is lessened so that cancer cells are not stimulated to grow.

There are a number of natural bioflavonoids that inhibit the activity of aromatase, and quercetin is one of them[8,9,10]. Although quercetin is not as potent as letrozole, it certainly has aromatase inhibition effects. At the end of the day the goal is to reduce the activity and the levels of estrogen as much as possible. Quercetin is a simple supplement that can be used together with conventional medications to achieve that goal.

One of the biggest challenges with quercetin is the bioavailability of the flavonoid. It tends to be very poorly absorbed when taken orally, making it difficult to achieve clinically relevant levels in the blood. It is possible to administer quercetin by intravenous therapy but some patients have significant sensitivity reactions to this. Quercetin however is very safe and well tolerated when taken orally. There are a number of professional supplement companies that have found solutions to this absorption problem.

If you expect to consume quercetin for its therapeutic effect, you need a high quality brand. Without the correct brand you will literally absorb nothing and you will not get the therapeutic effect. It is possible to enzymatically activate isoquercetin to make it more bioavailable and there is substantial evidence to indicate that this form is absorbed in the body at therapeutically relevant doses. Only a qualified Naturopathic doctor will be able to help you determine which is the right supplement for you.

Although quercetin is an antioxidant, at typical therapeutic doses it is not a strong enough antioxidant to interfere with chemotherapy. A bowl of blueberries would have a more substantial antioxidant effect than quercetin, and your oncologist should not be discouraging you from eating blueberries. Research indicates that with a select few chemotherapies, quercetin enhances the effectiveness of the chemotherapy while reducing side effects. For example, when cancer cells are pretreated with quercetin, the chemotherapy cisplatin is much more effective[3]. This effect is particularly pronounced with head and neck cancers. There is also evidence to suggest that it works synergistically with the chemotherapy Adriamycin when treating breast cancer cell lines.

Although quercetin can work synergistically with several chemotherapies, it is not universally safe with chemotherapy. Quercetin is an inhibitor of CYP2C8 which is the same pathway by which the chemotherapy paclitaxel is metabolized. This is a clear contraindication because it could potentially increase serum levels of the drug and lead to harmful side effects[1]. Quercetin should not be used during chemotherapy unless it is under the supervision of an experienced Naturopathic doctor.

EGCG

Epigallocatechin gallate (EGCG) is an extract from green tea that has shown great promise as an integrative cancer therapy. The mechanism of action is complicated because it interacts with multiple molecular pathways to inhibit the growth of cancerous cells. When cancer cells are exposed to EGCG, it triggers cell death by a variety of mechanisms[11,12,13,14]. Not only does it inhibit the growth of cancerous cells, but it also slows down the rate of metastasis.

One important characteristic of EGCG is that it acts as an anti-angiogenic substance. Angiogenesis is the growth of new blood vessels into a developing tumour. This process is necessary when cancer cells are spreading because the smaller growths need a blood supply to sustain their rapid growth. Cancer cells will often secrete chemicals that trick the human body into growing blood vessels into the tumour. EGCG helps to inhibit this process by inhibiting the viability of capillary tube formation and migration. This effect seems to be greatly enhanced by a new class of drugs called ERK inhibitors[12].

Tumour samples of mice treated with EGCG clearly show that the cancerous cells have reduced ERK activity while having enhanced p38 and JNK activity. In other words, the pathways that promote growth are down-regulated and the pathways that inhibit growth are up-regulated. The net effect is that the cancer does not grow or spread as quickly. Every molecular marker that was tested indicated that the cancer was less aggressive and more prone to cell death. If you perform a quick Google scholar search, you will see hundreds of well-controlled studies that consistently demonstrate this anti-cancer effect.

When EGCG is combined with curcumin at high doses, it helps to stabilize leukemias and lymphomas. There are many well-documented cases of patients with multiple myeloma who have had long-term disease stabilization by simply taking high doses of EGCG and curcumin. These natural compounds work synergistically to reduce inflammation and promote cell death in cancerous cells. The effectiveness of EGCG in multiple myeloma is undeniable, and this has resulted in a resurgence of research into its use as an adjunctive cancer therapy[16].

There are a handful of chemotherapy drugs where the use of EGCG is contraindicated such as Velcade (Bortezomib). There is contradictory information about the significance of this interaction, but it is still best to avoid combining EGCG with Velcade[15]. Some doctors focus on this one interaction while ignoring the overwhelming evidence that EGCG often acts synergistically with other forms of chemotherapy. It is difficult to argue against the use of EGCG if you take the time to actually look at the evidence. When EGCG is combined with cisplatin, it not only significantly increases the effectiveness of the drug, it also dramatically reduces the side effect profile[17,18,19].

This is another example of a supplement where the quality makes a significant difference. In order to obtain the desired anti-cancer effect, you must take high doses of quality EGCG. Drinking green tea can be helpful in the context of cancer prevention, but when it comes to cancer treatment, you need much higher doses. Some physicians recommend that patients get EGCG administered by intravenous therapy to get the doses as high as possible. The doses required to enhance chemotherapy and promote cell death in cancerous cells are quite high, but they are obtainable by consuming EGCG orally. It is also important to point out that this treatment is cost effective and generally well tolerated by patients.

Melatonin and Cancer

Everyone has heard about melatonin and how it can be used to promote restful sleep. Melatonin is a critical component of the circadian rhythm, and it is one of the molecular signals that tells our cells whether it is day or night. Every living organism on the planet has a circadian rhythm and our cells are strongly programmed around the day and night cycle. I have seen countless times where patients were prescribed melatonin by another Naturopathic doctor, but the patient discontinued it because they thought their sleep was fine. This suggests a misunderstanding between the patient and some of my colleagues regarding the reason for prescribing melatonin in the context of cancer. Whether the patient is sleeping well or not is secondary. They should be taking this supplement because of melatonin's potent anti-cancer properties.

Melatonin triggers cell death in cancerous cells and it has several properties that make it useful as an adjunctive cancer therapy[20,21,22]. The conclusion from a paper in the prestigious journal *Cancer Research* stated that:

Physiologic and pharmacologic concentrations of the pineal hormone melatonin have shown chemopreventive, oncostatic, and tumour inhibitory effects in a variety of in vitro and in vivo experimental models of neoplasia. Multiple mechanisms have been suggested for the biological effects of melatonin. Not only does melatonin seem to control development alone but also has the potential to increase the efficacy and decrease the side effects of chemotherapy when used in adjuvant settings. (Jung and Ahmad 9789)

There is also evidence to suggest that melatonin acts as a proteasome inhibitor and this could explain some of its anti-cancer effects[26]. The use of melatonin is particularly indicated in cases of estrogen positive breast cancer. For those who are taking tamoxifen or letrozole as a long-term therapy, it is certainly helpful to add melatonin into the treatment plan. The cancer prevention properties of melatonin appear to be mediated through the estrogen response pathway[29]. Recent research suggests that the development of breast cancer is linked to disruptions in the circadian rhythm. This could be one of the mechanisms by which melatonin halts the growth of cancerous cells.

When used appropriately, melatonin not only decreases side effects from chemotherapy, it also significantly enhances its effectiveness. In one randomized study, lung cancer patients were treated with chemotherapy alone or chemotherapy with melatonin. The melatonin group lived significantly longer with a reduced side effect profile[24]. This is just one example of many clinical trials. Melatonin can be used during chemotherapy or radiation, and the antioxidant effect is considered supportive of these conventional therapies[25].

In my experience, the high doses of melatonin (20mg) are well tolerated when they are used properly. The most common complaint that I hear from patients is that they feel groggy the next morning. Upon further questioning, it becomes clear that they did not use the melatonin correctly. You must take it before bed; but after you take the melatonin, you must avoid light! This means no television, no iPad's and no reading.

When light touches your eyes this inhibits the activity of melatonin. This makes sense considering how connected melatonin is to the circadian rhythm. Think about it for a second. A thousand years ago when our ancestors went to sleep, they would not have encountered light again until the sun rose. When you are exposed to light after taking melatonin, it sends mixed messages to your brain and disrupts the circadian cycle. This often results in a sensation of grogginess the next morning. It is critical that after you take melatonin, you immediately go into a dark room and sleep.

One other interesting note about melatonin is how its metabolic effects are easily disrupted by magnetic fields[23]. The clinical significance of this disruption is unclear, but this is not surprising given how delicate the circadian rhythm is. What is also interesting is that magnetic fields appear to disrupt the positive benefit from tamoxifen as well[27]. This does not mean that everyone should panic and avoid all sources of magnetic fields since this is virtually impossible to do in modern day society. The threshold for this inhibitory effect is not well established, however, it is worthwhile to point out this interaction. Perhaps people wanting to prevent cancer should reduce their exposure to excessive magnetic fields when possible[28].

Grape Seed Extract

This common cancer remedy is relatively unknown in the general population, yet it is well studied in the scientific community. Before discussing grape seed extract, it is very important to note that this is not the same as grapefruit. Grapefruit is contraindicated with chemotherapy as it directly interacts with the chemical pathways that break down chemotherapy. Grape seed extract is completely different, and it is associated with a number of anti-cancer effects.

Grape seed extract has been shown to significantly decrease the side effects from chemotherapy without reducing its effectiveness. It is an antioxidant that helps to eliminate free radicals before they damage healthy cells. Keep in mind that just because it is an antioxidant does not mean that it is contraindicated with chemotherapy. The broad generalization that all antioxidants should be avoided during chemotherapy is simply not supported by scientific evidence[30,31,32].

Grape seed extract is a weak antioxidant and you will certainly get more antioxidants from a balanced healthy diet. Antioxidants at very high doses are certainly contraindicated. But at normal doses these supplements can be supportive of chemotherapy. It protects healthy cells from damage much more than it protects the cancer cells.

When grape seed extract is combined with the chemotherapy doxorubicin, there is a potent synergistic effect against breast cancer cells[30]. Grape seed extract appears to inhibit the expression of VEGF by reducing HIF-1a protein expression[35]. In other words, grape seed extract is an anti-angiogenic substance because it inhibits the signal that cancer cells use to trick the body into growing blood vessels into the tumour. Inhibiting this blood vessel growth is essential to slow down both the growth and spread of cancer. When cancer cells are exposed to grape seed extract, their growth is halted and they undergo programmed cell death. This is similar to the effects of EGCG and these two natural supplements work well together.

There is a large body of evidence which indicates that grape seed extract is a potent natural aromatase inhibitor. This has significant implications for breast cancer and prevention of breast cancer post surgery. A recent study demonstrated a significant reduction in estrogen positive breast cancer recurrence in patients using doses of grape seed extract as high as 6g per day. This study was conducted on patients who did not tolerate letrozole or tamoxifen. Not only does grape seed extract significantly decrease the activity of aromatase, it also dramatically reduces the expression of aromatase. In other words, it stops cells from producing the enzyme in addition to inhibiting the actual activity of aromatase[33,34]. In my opinion every woman on anti-estrogen therapies to prevent recurrent breast cancer should also be on grape seed extract. It is a simple yet effective therapy that is extremely well tolerated by patients.

Indole-3-Carbinol

Indole-3-Carbinol (I3C) is a natural supplement that is useful in the treatment of both blood cancers and hormone dependent cancers. I3C is commonly found in cruciferous vegetables such as broccoli and cauliflower. It helps the liver to metabolize estrogen and break it down into a form which is less likely to promote the growth of hormone dependent cancers. There are many well-controlled studies in humans and animals which clearly demonstrates this anti-cancer effect.

Several animal studies have shown that when I3C is consumed, the animals are less likely to develop cancer when exposed to carcinogens. In other words, the I3C prevents the initiation of cancer. This same mechanism also applies to humans and is clinically significant. In one randomized study, patients with cervical intraepithelial neoplasia (CIN) were treated with I3C orally for 12 weeks. There was a statistically significant regression of CIN in the patients treated with I3C and the ratio of 2/16a hydroxyestrone changed in a dose dependent fashion[36].

In the past it was hypothesized that there were "good estrogens" and "bad estrogens" depending on how the hormone was metabolized. Preliminary research initially indicated that the 16a hydroxyestrone was the "bad estrogen" associated with promoting the growth of cancers. It was also thought that the "good estrogen" was the 2 hydroxyestrone. Early research also indicated that the ratio of 2/16a hydroxyestrone was indicative of cancer risk. Further analysis of this research indicates that a simple ratio does not give the complete clinical picture. What is clear is that therapies such as I3C encourage the metabolism of estrogen and have an anti-cancer effect. However, it seems that this effect cannot be attributed to a simple ratio of estrogen metabolites.

Research on the therapeutic mechanism of I3C has focused on estrogen metabolism, but there appears to be much more to this anti-cancer effect. I3C induces a G1 growth arrest in cancerous cells[37]. This is important because this is early in the cell cycle. This is the phase of the cell cycle where all the enzymes are made in preparation for cell replication. When a cancer cell is stopped at this phase in the cell cycle, it can significantly reduce the rate of growth. The exact mechanism of this cell cycle arrest is not fully understood, but it is thought to be linked to the inhibitory effect that I3C has on the transcription factor STAT3.

Recently there have been a number of supplement companies promoting the use of diindolylmethane (DIM), which is essentially the activated form of I3C. It is often promoted as being more potent because the body does not need to metabolize the I3C to make the "active ingredient" DIM. Although it is clear that many of the positive attributes of I3C can be linked to DIM, I do not believe that all of the positive effects can be linked to one metabolite of I3C. When the body metabolizes I3C, this produces numerous molecules and the cumulative effect of these metabolites is poorly defined.

There is always a push in medicine to find that one magical active ingredient. With this narrow focus we lose sight of the fact that all of these molecules serve a purpose even if we do not currently understand the mechanism. Although DIM can be an effective supplement, when it comes to cancer prevention I firmly believe that I3C is superior when used for long periods of time.

The bottom line is that I3C influences a number of different pathways that can inhibit the growth of cancerous cells. It is a useful tool for preventing the development of hormone dependent breast cancer after surgery. There is research to suggest that supplementation with I3C acts synergistically with tamoxifen[38]. In my clinical experience, it also tends to reduce the side effects that are all too common with anti-estrogen drugs. In my opinion this is a supplement that every person fighting a hormone dependent cancer should be on. It is safe and effective especially when used in conjunction with conventional therapies.

Reishi

Ganoderma lucidum (Reishi) is a medicinal mushroom that has been used in Asia for thousands of years to promote health and longevity. Only recently has science taken this ancient remedy seriously and investigated its anti-cancer potential. There are several obvious metabolic changes that occur in cancer patients who use reishi.

Many of the metabolic changes that occur with reishi are well-documented and understood in great detail. Reishi suppresses cell adhesion and cell migration of highly invasive breast and prostate cancers, thus reducing tumour invasiveness[39]. Consumption of reishi results in a powerful suppression of the transcription factors NfKb and AP-1, thus inhibiting uPA and its receptor uPAR. By influencing this pathway it has profound effects on the rate of growth and spread of cancerous cells. Reishi has clearly demonstrated anti-cancer activity in experimental models and in human trials. It appears that reishi suppresses the expression of several genes associated with cancer cell survival, including BCL-2, TERT and PDGFB[41]. This information is significant because conventional therapies will not be effective if the cancer cell is able to survive by modifying these pathways.

It is important to point out that reishi acts as an immune tonic. In other words, it does not stimulate the immune system but rather helps to balance it. This is particularly relevant to cancers that originate from the immune system such as lymphomas. In most cancers, the goal is to stimulate the immune system as much as possible so that the immune cells will attack the cancer more effectively.

In the case of lymphomas, many of the supplements that stimulate the immune system will also stimulate the cancer. This is because these specific cancer cells share a number of characteristics with the immune system where they originated. In these cases you must avoid supplements like astragalus and echinacea. Reishi however is still indicated for these cases because of its potent inhibition of NfKb and the fact that it protects the immune system without stimulating it.

Reishi is more effective when combined with conventional therapies. The evidence for its use as a stand alone therapy is debated, however, there is no debate about its effect as an adjunctive cancer therapy[40]. Higher doses of reishi are not necessarily more effective than moderate doses. When used at moderate doses, reishi is generally safe to use as an adjunctive cancer treatment.

Coriolus Versicolor

Coriolus versicolor is a fungus also known as turkey tail, which has received attention in the media as a potential cancer therapy. The medical community initially approached this remedy with skepticism, but it seems they have changed their tune after the isolation of a compound called Poly Saccharide K (PSK). Major medical centres such as MD Anderson have reported that, "it is a promising candidate for chemotherapy prevention due to the multiple effects on the malignant process, limited side effects and safety of oral dosing for extended periods of time."

PSK was initially isolated from turkey tail and there has since been a surge in research on its use as an adjunctive cancer therapy. It appears that much of the benefit of PSK is due to its effect on the immune system. PSK has been identified as a biological response modifier because it enhances the host versus tumour response. When patients are supplemented with PSK, it enhances the response of natural killer cells by influencing the release of cytokines in the body. There are also well-controlled studies which demonstrate that PSK inhibits the invasiveness of the cancer itself.

Turkey tail is most commonly used in conjunction with chemotherapy to support the immune system. There are several clinical trials which support the use of PSK in conjunction with chemotherapy. One large scale study conducted in 1992 showed a significant benefit to post menopausal breast cancer patients taking PSK in addition to chemotherapy[42]. More recent studies have indicated that it has significant potential with a wide range of cancers including colorectal, gastric, breast, liver, pancreatic and lung cancer. In Japan, PSK is used by Medical oncologists in conjunction with chemotherapy[43]. Due to its immune activating effects, PSK may not be safe to use with certain forms of lymphomas. The mechanism of action appears to be more related to immune stimulation, in contrast to reishi, which tends to balance the immune system.

New research is constantly coming out on PSK and its use in cancer. The conclusions of each study consistently demonstrate that this is a safe therapy which can be used in conjunction with chemotherapy to improve outcomes. In the near future, it is likely that the use of PSK will spread to conventional cancer clinics around the world.

Summary:

- The quality of your supplements makes a significant difference

- Micronutrient testing is not helpful in the context of integrative cancer care

- Quercetin inhibits cancer's ability to eliminate chemotherapy. It acts synergistically with some chemotherapies, but it is not universally safe with chemotherapy. Quercetin also acts as an aromatase inhibitor, which has significant applications in cancer prevention

- EGCG is found in green tea and at higher doses it helps to inhibit the growth of blood vessels into tumours. It is synergistic with the chemotherapy cisplatin

- Melatonin is not just useful for sleep. It is extremely helpful at reducing side effects from chemotherapy and it has potent anti-cancer properties

- Grape seed extract is a potent natural aromatase inhibitor that can significantly reduce the recurrence of hormone dependent cancers. It is synergistic with the chemotherapy doxorubicin

- Indole-3-Carbinol helps the body to metabolize estrogens and it can slow the rate of cancer proliferation. I3C works synergistically with tamoxifen

- Reishi balances the immune system and is particularly potent against lymphomas, breast and prostate cancers

- Coriolus versicolor stimulates the immune system and is particularly synergistic with several chemotherapies

References:

1. Bun, S. S., et al. "Drug interactions of paclitaxel metabolism in human liver microsomes." *Journal of chemotherapy* 15.3 (2003): 266-274.

2. Jeong, Jae-Hoon, et al. "Effects of low dose quercetin: Cancer cell-specific inhibition of cell cycle progression." *Journal of cellular biochemistry* 106.1 (2009): 73-82.

3. Sharma, Himani, Sudip Sen, and Neeta Singh. "Molecular pathways in the chemosensitization of cisplatin by quercetin in human head and neck cancer." *Cancer biology & therapy* 4.9 (2005): 949-955.

4. Scambia, G., et al. "Quercetin potentiates the effect of adriamycin in a multidrug-resistant MCF-7 human breast-cancer cell line: P-glycoprotein as a possible target." *Cancer chemotherapy and pharmacology* 34.6 (1994): 459-464.

5. Shapiro, Adam B., and Victor Ling. "Effect of quercetin on Hoechst 33342 transport by purified and reconstituted P-glycoprotein." *Biochemical pharmacology* 53.4 (1997): 587-596.

6. Zanini, Cristina, et al. "Inhibition of heat shock proteins (HSP) expression by quercetin and differential doxorubicin sensitization in neuroblastoma and Ewing's sarcoma cell lines." *Journal of neurochemistry* 103.4 (2007): 1344-1354.

7. Wei, Yu-quan, et al. "Induction of apoptosis by quercetin: involvement of heat shock protein." *Cancer Research* 54.18 (1994): 4952-4957.

8. Otake, Yoko, et al. "Quercetin and resveratrol potently reduce estrogen sulfotransferase activity in normal human mammary epithelial cells." *The Journal of steroid biochemistry and molecular biology* 73.5 (2000): 265-270.

9. Brueggemeier, Robert W., John C. Hackett, and Edgar S. Diaz-Cruz. "Aromatase inhibitors in the treatment of breast cancer." *Endocrine Society*, 2013.

10. Huang, Zeqi, Michael J. Fasco, and Laurence S. Kaminsky. "Inhibition of estrone sulfatase in human liver microsomes by quercetin and other flavonoids." *The Journal of steroid biochemistry and molecular biology* 63.1 (1997): 9-15.

11. Ahmad, Nihal, Sanjay Gupta, and Hasan Mukhtar. "Green tea polyphenol epigallocatechin-3-gallate differentially modulates nuclear factor κB in cancer cells versus normal cells." *Archives of Biochemistry and Biophysics* 376.2 (2000): 338-346.

12. Shankar, Sharmila, et al. "EGCG inhibits growth, invasion, angiogenesis and metastasis of pancreatic cancer." *Frontiers in bioscience: a journal and virtual library* 13 (2007): 440-452.

13. Hwang, Jin-Taek, et al. "Apoptotic effect of EGCG in HT-29 colon cancer cells via AMPK signal pathway." *Cancer letters* 247.1 (2007): 115-121.

14. Shimizu, Masahito, et al. "EGCG inhibits activation of HER3 and expression of cyclooxygenase-2 in human colon cancer cells." *Journal of experimental therapeutics & oncology* 5.1 (2004): 69-78.

15. Shah, Jatin J., Deborah J. Kuhn, and Robert Z. Orlowski. "Bortezomib and EGCG: no green tea for you?." *Blood* 113.23 (2009): 5695-5696.

16. Shammas, Masood A., et al. "Specific killing of multiple myeloma cells by (-)-epigallocatechin-3-gallate extracted from green tea: biologic activity and therapeutic implications." *Blood* 108.8 (2006): 2804-2810.

17. El-Mowafy, A. M., et al. "Novel chemotherapeutic and renal protective effects for the green tea (EGCG): role of oxidative stress and inflammatory-cytokine signaling." *Phytomedicine* 17.14 (2010): 1067-1075.

18. Davenport, Andrew, et al. "Celastrol and an EGCG pro-drug exhibit potent chemosensitizing activity in human leukemia cells." *International journal of molecular medicine* 25.3 (2010): 465-470.

19. Sarkar, Fazlul H., and Yiwei Li. "Using chemopreventive agents to enhance the efficacy of cancer therapy." *Cancer Research* 66.7 (2006): 3347-3350.

20. Hill, Steven M., and David E. Blask. "Effects of the pineal hormone mela-
    tonin on the proliferation and morphological characteristics of human
    breast cancer cells (MCF-7) in culture." *Cancer research* 48.21 (1988):
    6121-6126.

21. Blask, David E., Leonard A. Sauer, and Robert T. Dauchy. "Melatonin as
    a chronobiotic/anticancer agent: cellular, biochemical, and molecular
    mechanisms of action and their implications for circadian-based can-
    cer therapy." *Current topics in medicinal chemistry* 2.2 (2002): 113-132.

22. Jung, Brittney, and Nihal Ahmad. "Melatonin in cancer management:
    progress and promise." *Cancer Research* 66.20 (2006): 9789-9793.

23. Liburdy, R. P., et al. "ELF magnetic fields, breast cancer, and melatonin:
    60 Hz fields block melatonin's oncostatic action on ER+ breast cancer
    cell proliferation." *Journal of pineal research* 14.2 (1993): 89-97.

24. Lissoni, P., et al. "Five years survival in metastatic non-small cell lung
    cancer patients treated with chemotherapy alone or chemothera-
    py and melatonin: a randomized trial." *Journal of pineal research* 35.1
    (2003): 12-15.

25. Sanchez-Barcelo, Emilio J., et al. "Melatonin uses in oncology: breast
    cancer prevention and reduction of the side effects of chemotherapy
    and radiation." *Expert opinion on investigational drugs* 21.6 (2012): 819-
    831.

26. Vriend, Jerry, and Russel J. Reiter. "Melatonin as a proteasome inhibitor.
    Is there any clinical evidence?." *Life sciences* 115.1 (2014): 8-14.

27. Harland, Joan D., and Robert P. Liburdy. "Environmental magnetic fields
    inhibit the antiproliferative action of tamoxifen and melatonin in a hu-
    man breast cancer cell line." *Bioelectromagnetics* 18.8 (1997): 555-562.

28. Stevens, Richard G. "Electric power use and breast cancer: a hyptothe-
    sis." *Am. J. Epidemiol.;(United States)* 125.4 (1987).

29. Hill, Steven M., et al. "The growth inhibitory action of melatonin on hu-
    man breast cancer cells is linked to the estrogen response system." *Can-
    cer letters* 64.3 (1992): 249-256.

30. Sharma, Girish, et al. "Synergistic anti-cancer effects of grape seed extract and conventional cytotoxic agent doxorubicin against human breast carcinoma cells." *Breast cancer research and treatment* 85.1 (2004): 1-12.

31. Kim, Helen, et al. "Chemoprevention by grape seed extract and genistein in carcinogen-induced mammary cancer in rats is diet dependent." *The Journal of nutrition* 134.12 (2004): 3445S-3452S.

32. Kaur, Manjinder, Chapla Agarwal, and Rajesh Agarwal. "Anticancer and cancer chemopreventive potential of grape seed extract and other grape-based products." *The Journal of nutrition* 139.9 (2009): 1806S-1812S.

33. Kijima, Ikuko, et al. "Grape seed extract is an aromatase inhibitor and a suppressor of aromatase expression." *Cancer research* 66.11 (2006): 5960-5967.

34. Eng, Elizabeth T., et al. "Suppression of estrogen biosynthesis by procyanidin dimers in red wine and grape seeds." *Cancer research* 63.23 (2003): 8516-8522.

35. Lu, Jianming, et al. "Grape seed extract inhibits VEGF expression via reducing HIF-1α protein expression." *Carcinogenesis* 30.4 (2009): 636-644.

36. Bell, Maria C., et al. "Placebo-controlled trial of indole-3-carbinol in the treatment of CIN." *Gynecologic oncology* 78.2 (2000): 123-129.

37. Hsu, Jocelyn C., et al. "Indole-3-carbinol mediated cell cycle arrest of LNCaP human prostate cancer cells requires the induced production of activated p53 tumor suppressor protein." *Biochemical pharmacology* 72.12 (2006): 1714-1723.

38. Cover, Carolyn M., et al. "Indole-3-carbinol and tamoxifen cooperate to arrest the cell cycle of MCF-7 human breast cancer cells." *Cancer Research* 59.6 (1999): 1244-1251.

39. Sliva, Daniel. "Ganoderma lucidum (Reishi) in cancer treatment." *Integrative cancer therapies* 2.4 (2003): 358-364.

40. Jin, Xingzhong, et al. "Ganoderma lucidum (Reishi mushroom) for cancer treatment." *The Cochrane Library* (2012).

41. Martínez-Montemayor, Michelle M., et al. "Ganoderma lucidum (Reishi) inhibits cancer cell growth and expression of key molecules in inflammatory breast cancer." *Nutrition and cancer* 63.7 (2011): 1085-1094.

42. Toi, M., et al. "Randomized adjuvant trial to evaluate the addition of tamoxifen and PSK to chemotherapy in patients with primary breast cancer. 5-Year results from the Nishi-Nippon Group of the Adjuvant Chemoendocrine *Therapy for Breast Cancer Organization*." Cancer 70.10 (1992): 2475-2483.

43. Sun, Chen, et al. "Polysaccharide-K (PSK) in Cancer-Old Story, New Possibilities?." *Current medicinal chemistry* 19.5 (2012): 757-762.

Chapter 9

Intentions and Cancer

**"Your body hears everything
that your mind says."
- Naomi Judd**

When I was only 16 years old, I became well known in the healing community for helping rock and roll legend Ronnie Hawkins heal from terminal pancreatic cancer. More than 13 years later, he is still doing well and it is great to see him so vital after all these years. My understanding of energy and the ability to work with energy has evolved significantly over the last 14 years. I have had, and continue to have, incredible experiences with energy healing. These experiences ultimately helped me gain a deeper understanding of energy and how it can be applied in a clinical setting. In my opinion, energy healing and focused intentions are powerful tools that every patient should use.

Although energy healing resonates with me due to my personal experiences with energy, it does not resonate with everyone. This is important for family members to keep in mind when trying to help a loved one deal with cancer. Ultimately the treatment plan that is chosen needs to be one that resonates with the patient. Even if you truly believe in energy healing and you recommend a healer with nothing but the best intentions, it needs to be something that the patient is ready for in order to be effective.

If the patient is not ready for it then it is not helpful to force this treatment plan on them. It is critical that the patient be actively engaged with the healing process. In most cases, it is only when the patient is actively engaged in their own healing that you can expect to see significant results. When the patient is ready for energy healing, it can always be added into any protocol.

Everyday in my practice I see cancer patients who feel that there is a strong emotional source to their cancer. Patients will often be able to directly connect the formation of their cancer with a stressful event in their life. This is not an imaginary connection. There are biological reasons why emotional stress can trigger the formation of cancer.

Stress can cause cancer. It is important to recognize that this is not a hypothetical concept. It is a statement that is well supported by scientific evidence[8,9,10]. The link between cancer and stress is well established and is not debated by the scientific community. Still, many people are not aware of how significant this connection is and often it is disregarded by Medical doctors, despite the body of evidence.

There are many metabolic reasons why stress inhibits the immune system in its fight against cancer. Natural killer cells are essential in resisting the progression and metastatic spread of tumours once they have developed[11]. It is clear that the activity of these crucial cells decreases significantly with stress[12]. In other words, the cells that patrol your body looking for abnormal cells are less active when you are under stress.

A key component in the development of cancer is the mutation rate of DNA. Several studies have shown that cells are less efficient at repairing DNA damage when a patient is stressed. Patients who are depressed have less effective repair of damaged DNA compared to their less depressed counterparts[13]. This is significant because the mutations that drive the initiation and development of cancer are not repaired as effectively in a patient under stressful conditions.

In addition to the effects of stress on DNA repair, additional research has shown that apoptosis is inhibited by stress[14]. When a cell begins to turn cancerous, the cell will undergo what is called programmed cell death (also known as apoptosis). In other words, when a cell starts to get too abnormal it will destroy itself. This is one of the most fundamental defense mechanisms that our body has to fight the development of cancer. When this process is inhibited, then clearly the risk for developing cancer is higher.

The good news is that you can help your body fight cancer by reducing stress and focusing your intentions on healing. One of the most comprehensive intervention studies in cancer research evaluated the effects of stress management techniques, such as relaxation on cancer recurrence following removal of malignant melanoma[15]. Not only did the relaxed group experience reduced psychological distress, they also had more active immune systems than the control group not practicing relaxation.

A six year follow up of these patients showed a trend toward greater recurrence and higher mortality rates in the control group, compared to the relaxed group[8]. The bottom line is that patients who focus on reducing stress and focus their minds on healing not only have a better prognosis, they also have lower rates of developing cancer in the first place. Given what we know about the connection between immune function and stress, this conclusion is not surprising.

When fighting cancer it is essential that the patient use every tool at their disposal to increase the chances of a successful recovery. The immune system must be strong to fight off any serious disease. Our minds can dramatically influence how our cells respond to stress and this is intimately connected to the function of the immune system[17]. We all need to take control of our health and use this mind-body connection to our advantage. By reducing stress and focusing our minds on healing we will live longer and happier lives[16]. This is a powerful tool that we can all use to our advantage.

Cancer is a complex disease. In order to fight this disease it is necessary for patients to combine several therapies to increase the chances of success. Too often patients focus on seeking exotic and expensive therapies at distant clinics. Many of these protocols give patients a long list of supplements to take and in many cases these therapies are not specifically indicated for the type of cancer that the patient is dealing with. Patients frequently are quick to make changes to their diet and initiate a supplement protocol, however, they often neglect the power of the mind.

When someone is diagnosed with cancer they are often overwhelmed with information from health care professionals, family, friends and their own internet research. With this sudden change in priorities, patients get caught up in going from one appointment to the next and they forget about one of the most important healing tools of all; focused intentions. You must remember that regardless of which treatment plan you are using to fight cancer, at the end of the day it is your immune system that must destroy the cancer cells. Chemotherapy and radiation can certainly help to destroy a good portion of the cancerous cells but they will never eliminate all of them. It is your immune system that must ultimately kill any residual cells and clean up the debris.

Your cells will powerfully respond to the signals that they receive from your mind. By responding to these signals it allows your cells to more effectively adapt to the immediate environment. For example, if someone is about to jump off of a diving board and they are afraid of heights, just thinking about jumping will fundamentally change their cellular environment. This simple thought of jumping will cause the heart rate to elevate, the pupils to dilate and it will increase blood flow to muscles in the body.

At first this may seem like a counter productive response but it is a brilliant biological mechanism. The increased heart rate and blood flow to muscles allows the person to move faster during the act of jumping. The dilated pupils allow the person to see sharper images so that they can respond appropriately. The bottom line is that this simple intention about the immediate environment changed how every cell in that person's body reacted.

Your perception of your environment directly affects the biochemistry of your cells. This is a simple well established concept that can also be applied to healing. A positive and focused patient will have a stronger immune system compared to someone who is unfocused and negative.

Ultimately the goal when fighting cancer is to modify every possible lifestyle factor to enhance the strength of the immune system. The evidence clearly demonstrates that a stressed patient will have a significantly weaker immune system[1]. Patients must be actively encouraged to reduce stress and focus their intentions on healing. These simple mindful changes can make a substantial difference in the healing process.

Emotions and Illness

Over the past 14 years I have seen thousands of people with a wide range of serious illnesses. With the majority of these people, I immediately felt that there was a strong emotional component to their illness. Your cells store emotions and for this reason it is important to address these emotions which are inhibiting your healing. There is one experience which really stands out in my mind as a powerful illustration of the connection between emotions and illness.

When I was 16 I had the privilege of speaking at a First Nations healing gathering where there were many tribal elders in attendance. Several of these elders began to tell me heartbreaking stories from their past as many of them attended residential schools. Children were forcibly taken from their parents and placed into residential boarding schools where abuse was rampant. Many children died as a direct result of these horrible abuses. Their culture was decimated from the inside out, starting with the forced dismantling of the family unit. Some of these people were over 80 years old and they were brought to tears as they discussed their experiences at the residential schools.

Even though these terrible things happened to them almost 60 years ago, it still clearly affected them. They were deeply scarred on the emotional level and these scars have affected them on many different levels. They had physical ailments in their bodies where they felt that they stored these emotions. Aspects of their lives continue to be in chaos as a result of these past traumas. This had to have been a very traumatic event to bring a group of elders to tears about something that happened so long ago. It broke my heart to watch these elderly men and women break down about past events that were beyond their control.

There is absolutely no question that these past events were still influencing their health on emotional and physical levels. In order to heal a chronic illness, you must address the root cause of the problem. In this case these deeply-rooted emotions must be addressed if real healing is to occur.

It is important to remember that you are in complete control of your own emotions. Do not let emotions take control of you because you are the boss of your own cells. You know what is best for your cells so make sure that you create the ideal healing environment by changing your thought patterns accordingly. You must process through emotions rather than simply pushing the emotions aside. It is easy to push emotions to the background and pretend like it is not affecting you. This is not an effective way to heal on the emotional level. You must make an active effort to process through these different emotions. If an emotion is not processed then it lives within us. Time does not heal the wounds that occur in childhood. It simply conceals them. These deeply-concealed emotional wounds must be addressed in order to optimize the healing process.

We can certainly feel it in our bodies when we are overwhelmed by negative emotions. In some cases these emotional issues manifest into a serious physical ailment. Before this physical problem can be effectively treated, you must first address the underlying emotional source. The emotional and physical bodies are so interlinked that it is impossible to separate the two. You simply cannot influence one without influencing the other.

The physiology of emotions is a well-researched subject. When you are stressed there are "stress hormones" released from glands throughout your body. A well-known example of a stress hormone is cortisol. This hormone is released from the adrenal glands when your body is under stress. During stressful times your sympathetic nervous system (also known as the fight or flight response) is activated which stimulates the release of cortisol. Cortisol weakens the activity of the immune system by preventing the proliferation of T-cells. In other words, your immune system will not be as strong in the presence of this hormone because the cells that you need to fight the disease are not being activated. This pathway is so important that some bacteria deliberately stimulate the release of cortisol so that the immune system is weaker. This allows them to survive in the body.

Cortisol levels are easily influenced by a variety of factors. Sleep deprivation is associated with higher levels of cortisol. This is why it is essential to get enough sleep, especially when you are trying to promote healing. There is even a strong link between your cortisol levels and the length of your commute to work. If you regularly have a long commute, then you will have higher cortisol levels in your blood. This has been replicated many times in several different experiments[18].

Just as there are many factors that increase your stress hormone levels, there are several simple changes that you can make to your daily routine which will decrease them. Exercise, yoga, music and meditation are all techniques that have been shown to decrease stress hormone levels. It is essential that you put aside some time every day to reduce these stress hormones. Just doing a simple relaxing visualization on a regular basis will make a significant difference.

Intentions and Cancer

Not only is the chemical environment in your body more conducive to healing when you are in a relaxed state of mind, you will also feel better! In conventional medicine, there is still a tendency to restrict thinking to biochemical markers and dismiss anything else as "psychological". This could not be further from the reality of what health is. Our health is not based solely on the concentration of a few arbitrary chemicals in our blood. Of course these chemicals can serve as an indication of our health but doctors must also consider how the patient feels. If the patient feels better from a particular therapy but there is no significant change in the chemical markers, this is still a success.

It is not just "psychological" if the person feels better. If the person feels better then their cells are feeling better and biochemical changes have occurred within their body. Our tests cannot possibly cover every chemical. There are just a few "main" chemicals that are considered in any test. You cannot separate the mind and the body; you cannot influence one without influencing the other. How the patient feels is one of the most important markers of health.

If you have a stressful day here and there, do not worry about the physiological effects of this stress. Our bodies are capable of handling stressful conditions from time to time. Just think of the stress hormones involved when our ancestors were running away from predators. This only becomes a problem when there are chronic high levels of stress hormones in the body. Over time, chronic stress significantly increases the probability of developing a variety of pathologies including cardiovascular disease and cancer. These stress hormones also have some interesting properties with regards to memory. Cortisol cooperates with adrenaline to create memories of short-term emotional events. This is why you can recall stressful moments in your life so vividly. Often we can recall the intensity of every sense (touch, taste, smell, sight, sound) during these emotionally-charged events. These hormones have powerful effects on our physiology and we must keep their levels under control so that we are in control of our stress hormones; not the other way around.

Emotions do not have to hold you back from your healing process. They should be used to your advantage. Use your emotions to get you "fired up" and focused on changing your health. You can even incorporate positive emotional memories into your visualization routines. If you feel that your emotions are holding you back from optimal healing, then seek emotional support.

Counsellors can be helpful to organize your thoughts and process through your emotions. These treatments that address emotions should be initiated from the first day of treatment as they can help you to harness the power of your own emotions. The bottom line is that when you are mindful and proactive, you are in complete control of your emotions. Take advantage of this fact and use emotions to accelerate your healing process.

Mind-Body Connection

Anyone who reads about using intentions for healing will quickly find that there are many different modalities and each one uses a specific set of rules. It is essential when using intentions for healing that you use whatever resonates with you. If there is a concept or technique that does not make sense to you or does not resonate with you for whatever reason, then don't use that in your healing routine. Over the years I have been given advice from many different respected and well-known healers about rituals they think I should incorporate into my practice. I always respectfully listen to what they have to say, and I remain open to incorporating changes that resonate with me.

It can be helpful to try different healing modalities. With each modality take in concepts that make sense to you and disregard concepts that do not. Create a modality that is unique to you by incorporating the ideas that strongly resonate with you. You are a unique energetic being, so by doing this you will create a modality that is the best fit for you. One concept may powerfully resonate with someone else but that does not mean that it has to resonate with you. There is no right or wrong answer when it comes to energy healing; there are just different approaches (and solutions) to the same problem.

Some people have difficulty getting into that focused mental state that is required for optimal healing to take place. Practicing meditation is a great way to get better at bringing your mind into that relaxed yet focused state. When you are visualizing for the purpose of healing, only do this for as long as you can stay focused. If that is only for a couple of minutes then that's fine. There is no point carrying out these visualizations once you lose your focus. When your mind starts to wander, you are clearly not focused on the problem at hand.

Your visualizations do not have to be focused only on healing, as your intentions have influence beyond health. Make it a habit of putting aside a couple of minutes every night visualizing how you want your next day to go. This can be simply the intention to have a peaceful day. By just putting that intention out there of the perfect next day, the probability of that event manifesting becomes more likely. Do not spend time worrying about whether you are doing the visualization correctly or not. If you have the constant focused intent, that is enough. The more you practice visualizations the easier they become.

Encourage others to become involved with these visualizations as well. For instance, there are many people who like to get together to visualize healing the Earth. This is a great cause and collectively groups like this can make a significant difference. When you get enough people thinking along the same wavelength then major changes will happen. This is often referred to in literature as the tipping point or critical mass. Make sure that you spread the word about the power of intentions. It is important to make the distinction that this is not a strange new age concept, but rather these ideas are strongly supported by a body of scientific evidence[19].

Energy Healing and Cancer

As soon as someone hears the word healer or the phrase energy healing, they often have a preconceived idea about what that actually means. For those who consider themselves scientifically minded, often there is a visceral response to immediately classify this as a pseudoscience and disregard its use as a therapy. For others, they perceive it as a miracle cure with the expectation that the problem will suddenly vanish and they will leave in a state of perfect health. The reality is that energy healing is in between these polar opposite opinions. There is scientific evidence to support the use of energy healing as an adjunctive cancer therapy. It is not the only therapy that patients should use but it can certainly be an effective tool to support cancer patients and keep their immune systems strong.

Often before a cancer diagnosis the abnormal cells have already been mutating and growing for many years. When a problem has been developing for such an extended period of time it is often unrealistic to expect a sudden change in the condition. In fact, if all the cancer cells were to suddenly die this would likely be lethal to the patient as the cellular debris would overwhelm the liver and kidneys. The battle with cancer is a grind and over time it can wear patients down both emotionally and physically. It is essential to be patient with the healing process and keep your mind focused on healing.

The therapeutic goal with energy healing is to help focus the immune system and have it recognize the cancerous cells more effectively. During an energy healing the patient will focus on the problem area and use different techniques to communicate with their own cells. These techniques help to guide the immune system because often the biggest problem is that the immune system is not recognizing the cancer. Not only do your cells respond to your own focused intentions, they respond to the intentions of others. The healer, also using his or her intentions, will help to direct the flow of energy throughout the patient's body and this is often a relaxing experience. It is an excellent technique to release stress (physical or emotional) and get every cell focused on healing.

Acupuncture is an ancient technique that can be combined with energy healing to relieve stress and restore the flow of energy throughout the body. It is a well established therapy for reducing stress[2,3] and keeping the immune system strong. Energy healing is also effective at reducing stress[5] and it has been shown to improve the health of oncology patients both in and out of the hospital setting[4]. In all these studies patients who regularly used these therapies did significantly better than the placebo groups. Even if you take the argument that it is only placebo (which it clearly is not), people are getting better with these simple therapies. At the end of the day, that is the objective above everything else. Placebo works even if the patient knows that it is a placebo. It is almost as if the placebo gives their body permission to heal. When acupuncture and energy healing are combined and the patient has a focused mind[6,7] then this will keep the immune system strong and optimize the patient's chances of success.

Energy healing is such a powerful tool yet has no contraindications. I cannot think of any other integrative therapy where you can confidently say that it is safe to use with any other therapy. It is a simple tool that will work synergistically with any medical treatment. This is something that every patient with a chronic illness should be doing on a regular basis because it does make a positive difference.

Over the years I have seen many patients experience incredible positive reactions to energy healing. In the media it is these miraculous recoveries that seem to get the most attention. Although it is great that these cases bring more attention to the power of energy healing, these stories often focus on the wrong thing. The focus often revolves around the work of the energy healer rather than the patient.

The most significant aspect about energy healing is the fact that every patient in the world has the ability to influence their own healing with their own intentions. This is an innate healing tool that every person on the planet possesses. This healing tool should be the most significant part of any energy healing story in the media. When the media focuses on the healer, it results in patients looking externally for answers, when the most powerful healing tool of all resides within each of us. Although the healer certainly helped with these healings, it is the patients' innate healing abilities that continue the healing process. Regardless of the treatment used, at the end of the day the body needs to be able to heal itself.

The bottom line is that when fighting cancer you want to make every possible change to boost your immune system. If there was a pill that gave the same benefit as energy healing combined with a focused mind, you can bet that every cancer patient would be on this. What is so exciting about energy healing is that you don't even need a pill. You can harness this powerful tool using your own mind. This is an innate healing ability that we were all born with. Our cells are constantly responding to the signals that they receive from the mind. This simple connection is something that every patient should be using on a regular basis.

Fear and Cancer

There is no doubt about it; the diagnosis of cancer is scary, however, you cannot let this fear consume you. It is essential that you focus your energy on fighting the cancer and enjoying life. If you let fear take hold of you, your cells will not be ready to fight. In my experience, patients who enter treatment with fear do not respond as well as those who are focused and determined to overcome the cancer. In many cases it seems that patients are more fearful of the treatment than they are of the cancer itself. You must eliminate this fear and be ready to whole-heartedly embrace the treatment as your answer to this illness.

Patients who are unsure of chemotherapy often feel fearful after visiting the Medical oncologist. Even in cases where chemotherapy is clearly the patient's best option, they sometimes become overwhelmed with fear and avoid it. The oncologist will spend time during the visit going over the survival statistics and all of the potential side effects from the chemotherapy. In some cases the fear of the cancer completely consumes the patient, and it is challenging for them to know where to begin to eliminate the fear around the disease. In these circumstances, it is sometimes helpful to incorporate an alternative approach to addressing the cancer.

Some people like to visualize sending love to the cancer. At first this seems like a ridiculous idea to send love to the very disease that threatens your life. But this gentle approach can be helpful for some patients. Send love to the cancer and send this message to the cancerous cells: "You can live with me but just don't hurt me." This method can be a helpful first step when it comes to eliminating fear around a cancer diagnosis.

There is an emphasis in conventional medicine on giving patients accurate statistics about their prognosis. The patients are told to base their hope on these statistics and anything outside of this is considered false hope. This is a terrible way to present information to patients. Too often I see patients completely focused on the "expiry date" that they were given. Even if the results start to look more positive they have that date rigidly stuck in their mind. As the date approaches, they lose their will to fight and their health rapidly declines. In many of these cases, I am certain that the cancer would not have progressed so rapidly had they not been fixated on the "expiry date" that they were given.

Of course we need to be honest with patients and give them realistic expectations. Having said that, why do we need to base our hope on statistics? Hope is the variable that changes the statistics. When someone gives up hope this results in a rapid deterioration of health. It is very important for all health care practitioners to inform patients of their prognosis in a careful and deliberate manner without crushing their will to fight.

When you look at cases of spontaneous remission, there is one thing that many of these patients have in common. They saw the cancer as a summons for change, not with blame or fear. They embarked on a journey of self-discovery. By embarking on this journey, they learned more about the root cause of their illness and this allowed them to heal from within. Too often we look externally for the answer to our problems and we forget that the most powerful healing tool of all is within us. Every person on the planet has a powerful innate healing ability. We just need to make an effort to access it and maximize it. Use this healing tool to eliminate the emotional root cause of the illness.

Fear is a big killer in cancer patients and the mainstream medical community must recognize this. There should be consistent efforts to keep the patients strong on the emotional level and reduce the negative influence of fear. Patients should be encouraged to participate in their own healing process and integrate different modalities together that resonate with them. Fear should not be used to force patients to do any particular treatment while disregarding other therapies that could potentially benefit them.

Visualizations during Chemotherapy

Visualizations can be an effective tool to focus the mind and eliminate fear surrounding a treatment. I always recommend that my patients visualize the chemotherapy working more effectively while they are receiving the drug. The following is a visualization that you can use to enhance the chemotherapy treatments:

- During the infusion, see the chemotherapy move up the vein and towards the target area (Image 1).
- Visualize the chemotherapy surrounding and infiltrating the cancerous cells only while leaving healthy cells untouched. The drug becomes increasingly concentrated around the abnormal cells.
- See the cancer cells dying in the presence of the chemotherapy (Image 2).
- After the cancer cells have been destroyed see the immune system being drawn to the area. White blood cells migrate to the area of concern looking for any potential problem. These cells will attack and eliminate abnormal cells before they develop into a problem (Image 3).
- At the end of the visualization, see your cells in a state of perfect health with no sign of there ever being a problem. The only cells that remain in the area of concern are perfect healthy cells.

Image 1

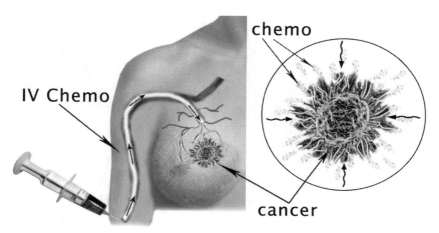

**See the chemotherapy move up the vein
and towards the target area.**

Image 2

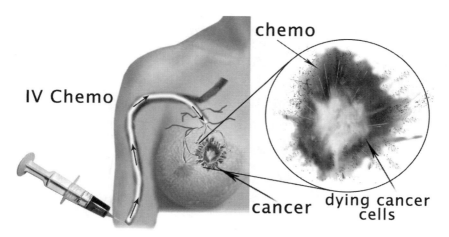

**See the cancer cells dying in the
presence of the chemotherapy.**

Image 3

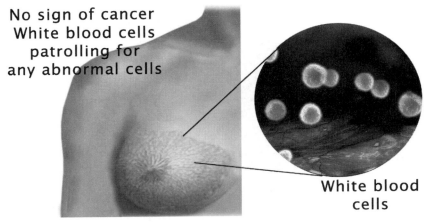

No sign of cancer
White blood cells
patrolling for
any abnormal cells

White blood
cells

**After the cancer cells have been destroyed see
the immune system being drawn to the area.**

This simple visualization should be done at every chemotherapy session and patients should be actively encouraged to do so. Not only will this help to control any fear of the treatment, it is a great exercise to keep your cells focused on the fight. Your cells respond powerfully to the signals from your mind and this is an excellent tool to keep the immune system strong in the area of concern.

Visualizations during Radiation

A similar visualization can also be used during radiation therapy. The most significant concern with radiation is that it may damage normal cells, thus increasing the chances of them transforming into cancerous cells. This concern can cause patients to be fearful of radiation treatments. The following is a visualization that you can use to enhance the radiation treatments:

- Visualize the radiation beam as being a precise laser. It passes through the normal tissues in your body without doing any harm. See the radiation beam hit the tumour and upon impacting the tumour it burns the abnormal cells. Only the tumour cells are affected and the normal tissues are left completely untouched (Image 4).
- See your immune system being drawn to the tumour like a magnet. White blood cells fill the area of concern and they immediately attack any residual abnormal cells.
- At the end of the visualization, there is no sign of the tumour and the only cells that remain are perfectly healthy cells (Image 5).

Image 4

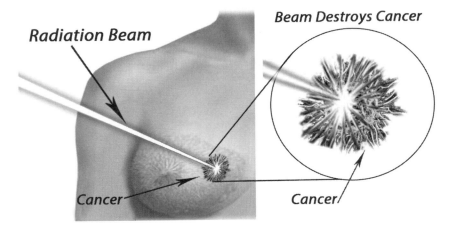

Radiation Beam

Beam Destroys Cancer

Cancer

Cancer

Visualize the radiation beam as being a precise laser. It passes through normal tissue in your body without doing any harm. See the radiation beam hit the tumour and upon impacting the tumour it burns the abnormal cells.

Image 5

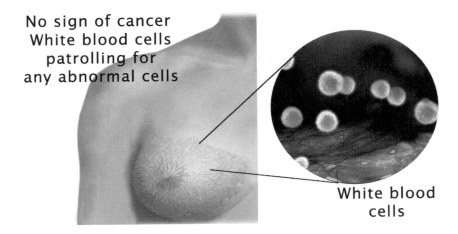

No sign of cancer
White blood cells
patrolling for
any abnormal cells

White blood
cells

With any visualization you can always modify it to be more targeted to the location of your cancer. Use whatever colour resonates best with you. At the end of your visualization, see your body in a state of perfect health with no sign of there ever being a problem. There are no firm rules to these visualizations and you can customize them however you want. In order to help patients visualize, I produced the DVD's: *Visualizations for Self-Empowerment* and *Heal Yourself*. These DVD's have numerous dynamic visualizations that can greatly assist patients with creating their own visualization routines. The vivid animations are useful tools for any patient who is interested in utilizing the mind-body connection for healing.

Too often we put the emphasis on physical treatments while forgetting about the power of the mind and the emotional health of the patient. A focused mind makes a significant difference with the healing process on both the physical and emotional levels. Patients need to be made acutely aware of the importance of visualizations in their healing process.

Spiritual Trips and Recharging Yourself

I am frequently asked by healers for advice on how to prevent them from burning out. Every patient that a healer sees will inevitably drain the healer's energy to some degree. There are conflicting opinions on this subject but the fact is that it takes energy to move energy. It is essential that every healer knows their own limit and takes the necessary time to recharge themselves. If you do not take time for yourself, you will eventually burn out and you will no longer be in a position to help others. In order to prevent burnout, find an activity that will help you recharge your own energy. Personally I find nothing recharges me better than a hike in the woods. The energy from the wilderness rapidly replenishes my energy.

I have been fortunate enough to have had the opportunity to travel to many spiritual locations across North America. One of the most interesting spiritual places that I have ever been to was Sedona. Sedona is approximately 100 miles north of Phoenix, Arizona. This small town is located in a desert valley with pillars of red rock scattered across the terrain.

I found it amazing that as I was hiking up steep hills in the scorching heat I did not feel drained at all. In fact I found that as I was climbing higher up I had more energy. As you hike up these unique rock formations there are plants that grow in strange ways. The branches appear to grow in a unique yet coordinated fashion forming distinct swirling patterns. Sedona is considered by many people to be one of the most spiritual locations in North America. It is rich with First Nations history and the unique landscape will remain engraved in my memory. I find that going to different spiritual locations helps to relax my mind and recharge my energy.

More recently I traveled to northern Nunavut with my father where we hiked the arctic tundra for several weeks. When my father was in his early 20's he worked on an icebreaker that went through these same areas. He told me stories of the ice being so thick that the 300 foot icebreaker actually got stuck for an entire day in the middle of the arctic summer. The terrain is now very different and you would not see such a large ship stranded in the now thin arctic ice. This northern adventure was something that I had wanted to do for many years and I am grateful that I had the opportunity to do so. This was a life changing experience that I will always remember.

The extreme seclusion of the arctic tundra was something that I had never experienced before. It was just me and my father with no sign of human civilization for many miles. As we looked at the rapidly changing glaciers it became immediately apparent how fragile these remote environments are. Even though there are no humans in sight, the effects of human civilization are clearly felt in these remote arctic regions. The glaciers are melting at an astonishing rate and it is amazing to see how much the terrain has changed even in the last ten years.

There was a unique beauty to this terrain that really resonated with me. The 24-hour sunlight was an interesting experience as it disrupted our natural circadian rhythms. This really changes your perspective on time because we are usually so dependent on having a night and a day. My father and I played a game where we tried to guess what time it was and it was amazing how clueless we were about the actual time. At one point we thought it was approximately noon but in reality it was three in the morning. At these northern latitudes, the sun does not rise or set in the summer. The sun rotates in small circles high in the sky. For me this arctic experience is my relaxing place. I like to visualize myself on a beach of the Arctic Ocean relaxing in the 24-hour sunlight and appreciating the beauty of the remote landscape.

When I am having trouble relaxing I like to picture myself being in these various relaxing environments. I highly recommend that you find a location that relaxes you. When you have such a place, you can easily put yourself there in your mind whenever you are feeling stressed. This will help to rapidly reduce your stress level and give your immune system the opportunity to restore balance. Even if you only place yourself in this relaxing environment for a few moments, it will help you significantly in your healing journey.

For myself I find that it is relaxing to go to one of these spiritual locations. Find a relaxing place in the wilderness away from the stress of every day life. Go for an invigorating hike in the woods. You must find time to get away and go to a calming place. By doing this it will help you unwind and recharge your energy. I cannot over emphasize the importance of this. If you do not take the time to recharge yourself then you will inevitably experience burnout.

As a teenager gifted in energy healing there was always a constant pressure to use my abilities to help someone in need. I was constantly being pulled in different directions towards people that were requesting my help. It took me a while before I learned to say no. It is difficult to tell someone that you cannot treat them, especially when they are in a terrible situation. Every healer needs to learn their own limit and this includes all health care professionals. We all have a limit to how much energy we can devote to helping others before we burn out. Sometimes you just need to stop and take time for yourself. When you are burnt out you won't be able to help anyone. In the long run, by taking such breaks and recharging yourself, you are able to help more people.

Summary:

- Focused intentions help to significantly reduce stress on your cells thus strengthening your immune system in the fight against cancer

- Energy healing and acupuncture are excellent techniques to utilize the mind-body connection and focus your cells on healing

- Often the biggest challenge for your immune system when fighting cancer is the recognition of which cells are healthy and which are not. By utilizing the mind-body connection you are sending a message to your cells that this is where they need to focus

- It is essential to eliminate the fear surrounding cancer and the associated treatments

- Visualize on a daily basis to stimulate the immune system, and see the treatments being more effective at killing the abnormal cells

- At the end of every visualization, you want to see yourself in a state of perfect health with no sign of there ever being a problem

- Do not base your hope on the statistics. Hope is the variable that changes the statistics

References:

1. Segerstrom, Suzanne C., and Gregory E. Miller. "Psychological stress and the human immune system: a meta-analytic study of 30 years of inquiry." *Psychological bulletin* 130.4 (2004): 601.

2. Middlekauff, Holly R., et al. "Acupuncture inhibits sympathetic activation during mental stress in advanced heart failure patients." *Journal of cardiac failure* 8.6 (2002): 399-406.

3. Hollifield, Michael, et al. "Acupuncture for posttraumatic stress disorder: a randomized controlled pilot trial." *The Journal of nervous and mental disease* 195.6 (2007): 504-513.

4. Cuneo, Charlotte L., et al. "The effect of Reiki on work-related stress of the registered nurse." *Journal of Holistic Nursing* 29.1 (2011): 33-43.

5. Shore, Adina Goldman. "Long-term effects of energetic healing on symptoms of psychological depression and self-perceived stress." *Alternative therapies in health and medicine* 10.3 (2003): 42-48.

6. Kox, Matthijs, et al. "The influence of concentration/meditation on autonomic nervous system activity and the innate immune response: a case study." *Psychosomatic medicine* 74.5 (2012): 489-494.

7. Morgan, Nani, et al. "The effects of mind-body therapies on the immune system: meta-analysis." *PloS one* 9.7 (2014): e100903.

8. Bovbjerg, Dana H. "Psychoneuroimmunology. Implications for oncology?." *Cancer* 67.S3 (1991): 828-832.

9. Spiegel D, Kato PM. Psychosocial influences on cancer incidence and progression. Harvard Rev Psychiatry 1996; 4: 10-26.

10. Andersen, Barbara L., et al. "Stress and immune responses after surgical treatment for regional breast cancer." *Journal of the National Cancer Institute* 90.1 (1998): 30-36.

11. Herberman RB. Immunotherapy. In Lenhard RE Jr, Osteen RT, Gansler T (eds): Clinical Oncology. Atlanta, GA: *American Cancer Society* 2001; 215-223.

12. Zorrilla, Eric P., et al. "The relationship of depression and stressors to immunological assays: a meta-analytic review." *Brain, behavior, and immunity* 15.3 (2001): 199-226.

13. Kiecolt-Glaser, Janice K., et al. "Distress and DNA repair in human lymphocytes." *Journal of Behavioral Medicine* 8.4 (1985): 311-320.

14. Tomei, L. David, et al. "Psychological stress and phorbol ester inhibition of radiation-induced apoptosis in human peripheral blood leukocytes." *Psychiatry research* 33.1 (1990): 59-71.

15. Fawzy, Fawzy I., et al. "Malignant melanoma: effects of an early structured psychiatric intervention, coping, and affective state on recurrence and survival 6 years later." *Archives of General Psychiatry* 50.9 (1993): 681-689.

16. Fawzy, Fawzy I., et al. "A structured psychiatric intervention for cancer patients: I. Changes over time in methods of coping and affective disturbance." *Archives of General Psychiatry* 47.8 (1990): 720-725.

17. Veenhoven, Ruut. "Healthy happiness: Effects of happiness on physical health and the consequences for preventive health care." *Journal of happiness studies* 9.3 (2008): 449-469.

18. Evans, Gary W., and Richard E. Wener. "Rail commuting duration and passenger stress." *Health psychology* 25.3 (2006): 408.

19. Hagelin, John S., et al. "Effects of group practice of the transcendental meditation program on preventing violent crime in Washington, DC: Results of the National Demonstration Project, June--July 1993." *Social Indicators Research* 47.2 (1999): 153-201.

Intentions and Cancer

Chapter 10

Cancer Prevention

"An ounce of prevention is worth a pound of cure."
- Benjamin Franklin

One of my first patients was a woman very fearful about the recurrence of cancer. She had a successful surgery and based on all the information that we had, she was cancer free. I would regularly receive emails from her asking about various supplements that she could use to prevent recurrence. It was obvious that she was consumed with fear and anxiety about the possibility of her cancer returning. When I discussed my concern with her and suggested that she consider counselling she immediately became defensive. She refused to accept that there was a significant emotional connection to her cancer. The fact that she was denying this connection spoke volumes considering how obviously these emotions were effecting her physically.

A comprehensive prevention plan was developed and she was following it diligently. The problem was that she was adhering to this plan out of fear. It was the fear of recurrence that was forcing her to do these treatments. I repeatedly tried to convince her to seek emotional help but she refused. Six months later she got another PET scan and her worst fears had manifested physically. A small mass was discovered close to the surgical site and upon hearing this news, she was devastated. At this point in time, the cancer is stable; however, the constant fear and anxiety continues to be a real challenge for this patient.

I always wondered whether her fear was due to her body recognizing the presence of cancer, or if the fear actually manifested the cancer. Your body is always sending you signals. You just have to listen to the messages that it is sending to you. It is entirely possible that this patient's body knew the cancer was there and the signal that it sent manifested as fear. My gut feeling is that there may have been some dormant cells in the area that were stimulated by this patient's fear. To this day I firmly believe that her clinical course would have been different had she focused on actually working through these emotions. We put too much emphasis on physical therapies when often the most important factor for cancer prevention is addressing the emotional root causes of the illness.

When you fear something, you are unintentionally giving energy to it. From a biological perspective, when you are in a state of fear your immune system will not be as effective. This subtle immunological shift can sometimes create an environment for dormant cancer cells to become active.

When a patient is told that their cancer was cured by a successful surgery, they should not suddenly stop integrative cancer therapies. After a successful surgery, you must continue to be treated as if there is an active cancer for the next year. Even with good surgical margins, it is possible that abnormal cells still remain. Cells get progressively more abnormal when they are in close proximity to a tumour. This is due to the fact that cancer dramatically changes the chemistry of its local environment.

Cells near the environment of the tumour are often metabolically abnormal and with the right conditions, they can turn cancerous. It is for this reason that you must keep the immune system strong and focused on addressing any remaining abnormal cells. This includes sticking to the positive changes made to your diet along with targeted supplementation that keeps your immune system strong. You must use every tool at your disposal to prevent the recurrence of cancer. The first year after surgery or chemotherapy is a critical time period where you must stay focused!

The mainstream medical community is slowly beginning to put more of an emphasis on preventative medicine. I find it interesting that governments are consistently speaking about the importance of preventive medicine, yet little is actually being done to prevent the development of chronic disease. Many patients get access to their primary physician through a walk-in clinic thus they will see a different Medical doctor every time they need medical attention. If you were to go to a walk-in clinic and tell the doctor, "I have nothing wrong, but I would like to be proactive and take steps to reduce my risk of developing disease," what do you think the response would be? I suspect that the feedback would be limited and the underlying message would be something along the lines of "stop wasting my time."

Our health care system needs to change so that it is normal for patients to seek help for prevention of illness rather than waiting until they have symptoms before seeking help. Naturopathic doctors can play a huge role in this preventative health care model. It is essential for patients to have a Naturopathic doctor who takes the time to go through their entire health history. By doing this, it is possible to develop a treatment plan that can help to prevent the development of disease.

Exercise and Cancer

Everyone has heard that exercise is good for your well-being. Exercise has been shown to elevate your mood and increase energy levels. Patients who regularly exercise are statistically less likely to develop a number of serious health conditions. The effectiveness of exercise is not questioned in the medical community; yet when it comes to cancer care, patients often forget about the benefits of exercise. Instead, they focus their attention on more exotic treatment plans. Exercise is not a cure for cancer but it is certainly an important part of any integrative cancer program.

How does exercise benefit cancer patients? There are many different reasons why exercise has such a positive impact on cancer patients. The immune system becomes more active during exercise as the monocytes increase the concentration of specific receptors on their surface[1]. Exercise also significantly helps patients with their sleep and it is well documented that the majority of healing takes place during sleep. When you get better quality sleep, your cells will be less stressed and this will significantly boost the strength of your immune system.

The mitochondria provide every cell in your body with energy required for any activity. During exercise, the mitochondria are stimulated to provide cells with sufficient energy for the activity. It is beneficial in the context of cancer to stimulate mitochondria, because the survival of cancerous cells is dependent on shutting down the mitochondria. The mitochondria reside within every cell in the body and they are normally the primary source of energy. In cancer cells the mitochondria are dormant and they are not the primary source of energy. Cancer cells deliberately make this metabolic shift because if the mitochondria were active they would immediately recognize that the cell in which they reside is abnormal.

When the mitochondria detects that the cell is abnormal, it will immediately trigger programmed cell death. In other words, if the mitochondria detects that the cell in which it lives is abnormal, it kills the cell. This is why cancer keeps the mitochondria dormant but exercise increases the chances of waking up the mitochondria. If more mitochondria are active, then there is a greater chance that the cell will undergo programmed cell death. The bottom line is that there are numerous physiological and psychological changes that occur with regular exercise which are very beneficial to cancer patients[3].

Several studies clearly demonstrate that patients undergoing chemotherapy or radiation do much better if they are exercising regularly[2,4]. Exercise is well documented to improve energy levels in patients and this is especially important for patients undergoing cancer treatment. One of the biggest challenges with patients during conventional cancer therapies is fatigue and a decreased sense of vitality. Exercise improves these common side effects.

Patients who regularly exercise during these therapies have better clinical outcomes and significantly improved quality of life. Although this is well established in the medical community, exercise is rarely suggested by Medical oncologists. This attitude needs to change because when the body is being exposed to toxic treatments, it is essential to use every tool at our disposal to help the body adapt to this stress. Exercise is an effective and basic tool which can help patients deal with the stress of chemotherapy and radiation.

Not only is exercise important during cancer therapies, it is also effective at preventing cancer recurrence[7]. Although some researchers dispute the significance of recurrence prevention, no one disputes that regular exercise decreases overall mortality in cancer survivors[5,6]. Women with estrogen positive breast cancer after a successful surgery will be put on tamoxifen for a minimum of five years to reduce the risk of recurrence by only a few percentage points in some cases[8].

In one large study of women with a history of breast cancer, it showed that women who walked three to five hours per week were 43% less likely to develop recurrent breast cancer and 50% less likely to die from breast cancer. This exercise group was compared to women who engaged in less than one hour of physical activity per week[9]. This study clearly demonstrates the importance of exercise in the context of cancer prevention. I find it amazing that some patients will readily comply with taking a drug for five to ten years, yet are resistant to regular exercise.

The exercise program does not need to be an extreme and rigorous routine, nor does it have to be a specific activity to prevent recurrence. All that matters is that your cardiovascular system gets a good workout from regular aerobic activity. Even a moderate cardio workout for less than 30 minutes, five days per week, can be very helpful. Make the time for this activity because it can make a significant difference in your response to treatment.

The bottom line is that at every phase in cancer treatment, regular exercise is a powerful adjunctive therapy. Regular exercise helps to prevent the development of cancer and it also helps patients to get through the aggressive cancer therapies necessary to kill cancer. More cancer patients need to be aware of the simple fact that regular exercise makes a significant difference when fighting cancer. This is a simple yet effective adjunctive therapy that should be actively encouraged in every patient capable of regular exercise.

Anti-Estrogen Therapies and Breast Cancer

After breast cancer has been surgically removed, it is common for patients to be put on either tamoxifen or letrozole for a minimum of five years. Recent research indicates that there is an increased benefit when patients are on the medication for a 10-year period. These therapies essentially work by reducing the production or biochemical effect of estrogen. These drugs can cause significant side effects, and many patients struggle to stay on the medication for the entire ten year period.

The good news is that there are many natural therapies that can be used to enhance the effectiveness of anti-estrogen therapies while reducing side effects. Grape seed extract was described in detail in chapter 8 (*Natural Supplements and Cancer*). There is no question that grape seed extract is a powerful natural aromatase inhibitor that works synergistically with anti-estrogen therapies to reduce the risk of recurrence. In my opinion, every woman on anti-estrogen therapy should also be on grape seed extract. High quality omega-3's in my clinical experience also seems to help substantially with the side effects of anti-estrogen therapies. The quality and the dose of omega-3's must be adequate because when lower doses are used, these benefits are generally not seen.

One factor that must be considered when choosing your strategy to prevent breast cancer recurrence is how estrogen positive your cancer is. Often patients are simply told whether it is estrogen positive or not, but this information is incomplete. There is a range of how sensitive the cancer is to estrogen and this makes a tremendous difference when choosing the appropriate strategy. The most commonly used scale is called the Allred score and it is measured out of eight. If it is zero out of eight then it is considered estrogen negative. If the test is 8/8, then this indicates that the cancer will respond strongly to estrogen. Anything over zero can potentially be considered positive (depending on the lab doing the test).

If the cancer is weakly estrogen positive, then the benefits of anti-estrogen therapies are minimal. In fact some oncologists will not recommend these therapies in these circumstances because the risks of the medication outweigh the potential benefits. Other oncologists tend to prescribe the medication even if the cancer is barely estrogen positive, despite the weak evidence to support its use. If the cancer is strongly estrogen positive (anything over a five), then the use of anti-estrogen therapies is certainly warranted.

In triple negative breast cancer the cancer cells will continue to grow even without estrogen. This type of cancer is much more challenging to deal with because there is no defined molecular target. A cancer that is strongly estrogen positive will grow much more rapidly in the presence of estrogen. If the estrogen is eliminated (or strongly reduced) with the medication, then the cancer will not grow as aggressively. Patients in these situations need to recognize that the estrogen is an excellent molecular target. If possible you should certainly target estrogen, because in these circumstances we know it will significantly reduce the risk of recurrence. Patients should also adhere to a healthy lifestyle and diet to reduce the risk of recurrence even more.

The bottom line is that if you have a strongly estrogen positive cancer, then the use of an anti-estrogen therapy is certainly indicated. Patients in this situation should give these prescriptions a good try and make a strong effort to stay on the drug for a minimum of five years. There are some patients who simply cannot tolerate any of the conventional medications, and in these circumstances there is a natural option. Ideally it is always best if patients are able to combine these different therapies rather than avoiding the conventional medications. However, in those who cannot tolerate the conventional drugs at all, I would recommend consuming high doses of grape seed extract.

The grape seed extract should be high quality and it should be taken at high doses (at least 2 grams per day). This natural approach should be considered a long-term therapy, just like the anti-estrogen therapies. It is not something that you experiment with for a few months and then discontinue. You need to consider this a long-term therapy that you continue for a minimum of five years. Ideally you would continue this therapy for ten years to optimally reduce the risk of recurrence.

If you are given the diagnosis of estrogen positive cancer, make sure that you ask the appropriate questions. You need to know how estrogen positive it is and get statistics based on this information. After getting these statistics, you can then make an informed decision about which therapeutic option is most appropriate for you. Often the best approach is combining multiple therapies and lifestyle changes to reduce the risk of recurrence as much as possible.

Diet and Cancer Prevention

A quick search on the internet will reveal hundreds of different diets that all claim to be the most effective at killing or preventing cancer. The reality is that there is no single diet that has been shown to be the most effective at fighting cancer. This topic was discussed in more detail in the chapter 2 (*Diet and Cancer*) and there are some situations where specific diets are certainly indicated.

In my clinical experience I have found that many of the dietary recommendations patients get from the internet or friends are completely inaccurate. Some health care practitioners who do not regularly work with cancer also tend to give dietary suggestions which are simply not practical in an oncology setting. You must develop a plan that you can realistically maintain for the rest of your life. Think about that for a second. We are not talking about a diet plan that you adhere to for a six week period. We are talking about a treatment plan that will last for the rest of your life.

Adhering to a diet plan on a short-term basis generally has no benefit in the context of cancer. The key to developing an effective long-term plan is to simply avoid the foods that are obviously harmful while introducing a few foods that are healthier choices. I realize that this sounds too simple but it is the best way to develop an effective and enjoyable long-term diet plan. A strict diet plan where the joy of eating is far removed is not necessarily more effective. It is difficult to quantify the positive effect that eating a food which you enjoy has on your body. I am sure that it makes a difference in the healing process, and I encourage patients to eat foods that they enjoy as long as it is not a significant contraindication.

In most cancer prevention diet plans, the foods that should be avoided are simple carbohydrates and red meat. The reasons for this are clearly described in chapter 2 (*Diet and Cancer*). Simply avoiding those two items should take priority over any other dietary change. Although these recommendations are the most important, you can develop a more specific cancer prevention diet based on your family history. If you have a family history of a specific type of cancer then you should tailor your diet plan to specifically address the relevant organ systems. Keep in mind that if you have some genes that are associated with an increased cancer risk this does not mean that you are destined to develop cancer. There are many factors that influence the development of cancer and genetics is only one of them. In my opinion the environment and diet are more important because these factors ultimately determine the expression of your genetics.

If you have a family history of colon cancer then it would be advisable to increase your intake of fibre. There are several external and internal toxins that significantly affect the health of the colon. Many foods including red meat get metabolized in the gastrointestinal tract in such a way that they become toxic when they reach the colon. Even some chemicals released by your own bodily fluid (bile from the gallbladder) will be metabolized by bacteria in the intestines to form cancer-causing compounds.

The good news is that when you consume more fibre, these toxins will bind to the fibre and be more effectively eliminated with each bowel movement. This removes the toxins before they have a chance to damage cells in the colon. Anyone with a family history of colon cancer should look for ways to add healthy amounts of fibre into their diet. It is essential to have adequate amounts of insoluble fibre as it not only helps to eliminate toxins but it also helps to control blood sugar levels.

Although it is challenging to find evidence to support this concept I firmly believe that there is a benefit to eliminating foods that you are sensitive to. There are several tests that can be done to determine your food sensitivities. The most accurate tests require blood work and I would not recommend basing these long-term decisions on muscle testing results. The proper tests involve getting a sample of blood and testing the blood for antibodies against various food antigens. The test will give you a digital printout showing a list of foods to which you reacted. When patients consume foods they are sensitive to, they often experience a wide range of symptoms such as fatigue, headaches, bloating, gas and abdominal discomfort.

When the body is regularly exposed to these foods that are causing low-grade inflammation, often the person is completely unaware of the problem. This makes sense because these patients are in a state of chronic inflammation and as far as their cells are concerned, this is a normal state. It is not until after these inflammatory foods are eliminated for a minimum of three months that this inflammation actually subsides. It is essential that you completely eliminate the inflammatory foods during this elimination period. Every time that you are exposed to the food, it will trigger inflammation and you are starting back at square one.

After this period of complete elimination the patient can then slowly reintroduce some of these foods. When the food is reintroduced, the patient should experience symptoms from the inflammation. These symptoms can be quite vague including (but not limited to) fatigue, bloating, discomfort or mind fog. This reintroduction test is the only way to really know for sure if you are sensitive to a food. If you experience any of these symptoms after reintroducing a food, then this likely means that the food is triggering inflammation. Obviously if a food is triggering inflammation then you should continue to avoid it.

Please do not attempt to do this elimination diet on your own. You must have professional guidance through this process. If you do not do it properly, then you will never know if you are truly sensitive to a food or if you simply carried out the process incorrectly. Any experienced Naturopathic doctor will be able to walk you through this elimination and reintroduction process. This can help you to identify several unique foods that you may be sensitive to. The bottom line is that if you are sensitive to a food, consumption of that food will trigger inflammation throughout your body. With professional guidance it is possible to properly identify these foods and eliminate this clear source of inflammation.

Mitochondrial Support and Cancer Prevention

The mitochondria are within every cell and they are critical to cellular survival. Often when the body is under stress, the mitochondria within cells are also stressed. There is a strong connection between mitochondrial dysfunction and the development of chronic disease. Cancer cells are dependent on mitochondrial dormancy. If the mitochondria were fully functional and healthy then the cancerous cell would undergo programmed cell death. Supporting the mitochondria with the necessary nutrients can help to maintain the health of all cells and prevent chronic disease.

The good news is that the scientific community has a deep understanding of how the mitochondria function. In the early 20th century it became apparent that the mitochondria are necessary for the generation of energy within mammalian cells. By the 21st century, research started to recognize the connection between mitochondrial metabolism and cancer[10,11,12,13]. Any treatment plan that attempts to prevent the development of chronic disease should make a strong effort to support mitochondrial health.

Although there are no large double-blind trials to support this hypothesis, there is an abundance of evidence and it is not hard to connect the dots. If your mitochondria are healthier, then your cells are healthier and you are less likely to develop disease. The mitochondria have been extensively studied and there are many well documented natural therapies that support mitochondrial health. The health of the mitochondria is quantifiable which makes it easy to assess the effectiveness of these natural treatments.

One of the most effective supports of mitochondrial health is aerobic exercise. When you exercise the energetic requirements for your cells increases. As a result, the mitochondria become more active in order to supply the cells with adequate energy. It is thought that many of the observed benefits of exercise are related to its influence on mitochondrial metabolism. This activation of the mitochondria keeps them healthy and it supplies every cell with the energy necessary to heal. Regular aerobic exercise is an integral component of any mitochondrial support plan.

Pyrroloquinoline quinone (PQQ) and coenzyme Q10 (CoQ10) are synergistic nutrients that support mitochondrial function. Supplementation with CoQ10 increases the efficiency of mitochondrial ATP production and cellular respiration[16,17]. PQQ has been shown to reduce oxidative stress on mitochondria while stimulating mitochondrial biogenesis[14,15]. In other words, when these molecules are taken together, it promotes mitochondrial health and the growth of new mitochondria within cells. These simple mitochondrial supports are neuroprotective, making them particularly indicated in neurodegenerative diseases.

Other mitochondrial supports include acetyl-L-carnitine (ALC), R-alpha lipoic acid (ALA), resveratrol and grape seed extract. ALC and ALA work synergistically to prevent mitochondrial decay[18]. Resveratrol is a natural antioxidant that is found in wine and it is well established as a stimulator of mitochondrial respiration in muscle tissue[19]. Grape seed extract is also a natural antioxidant that has been shown to improve mitochondrial function in muscle cells[20]. It is clear that there are many natural treatments that can be used to effectively support the mitochondria. The applications of mitochondrial support extend far beyond cancer. It has powerful implications for the aging process itself.

Taking large doses of these natural supports is not necessarily beneficial. A balanced mitochondrial support using the lowest doses possible would be better suited as a long-term plan. Future research will establish optimal dosing and combinations of these simple natural therapies. To keep our cells strong and prevent disease we need to go back to biology basics. If the mitochondria are healthy, then your cells will have the energy necessary to heal. If your cells are more effective at healing, then you are less likely to develop chronic disease.

Summary:

- Avoid simple sugars and red meat
- Avoid foods that are inflammatory to you
- Modify your lifestyle to address organ systems that are vulnerable based on your family history (eg. adequate fibre intake in patients with a family history of colon cancer)
- Exercise on a regular basis to enhance your immune system and promote a healthy cardiovascular system
- Support mitochondrial health with exercise and targeted supplementation to reduce the risk of developing chronic disease
- Meditate and visualize on a daily basis to reduce stress and stimulate the immune system

References:

1. Peters, C., et al. "Exercise, cancer and the immune response of mono-cytes." *Anticancer research* 15.1 (1994): 175-179.

2. Mock, Victoria, et al. "Effects of exercise on fatigue, physical function-ing, and emotional distress during radiation therapy for breast cancer." *Oncology nursing forum*. Vol. 24. No. 6. 1997.

3. Burnham, Timothy R., and Anthony Wilcox. "Effects of exercise on phys-iological and psychological variables in cancer survivors." *Medicine & Science in Sports & Exercise* (2002).

4. Courneya, KERRY S. "Exercise in cancer survivors: an overview of re-search." *Medicine and Science in Sports and Exercise* 35.11 (2003): 1846-1852.

5. Irwin, Melinda L., et al. "Randomized controlled trial of aerobic exercise on insulin and insulin-like growth factors in breast cancer survivors: the Yale Exercise and Survivorship study." *Cancer Epidemiology Biomarkers & Prevention* 18.1 (2009): 306-313.

6. Irwin, Melinda L., et al. "Influence of pre-and postdiagnosis physical ac-tivity on mortality in breast cancer survivors: the health, eating, activ-ity, and lifestyle study." *Journal of clinical oncology* 26.24 (2008): 3958-3964.

7. Loprinzi, Paul D., et al. "Physical activity and the risk of breast cancer recurrence: a literature review." Oncology nursing forum. Vol. 39. No. 3. *Oncology Nursing Society,* 2012.

8. Early Breast Cancer Trialists' Collaborative Group. "Relevance of breast cancer hormone receptors and other factors to the efficacy of adjuvant tamoxifen: patient-level meta-analysis of randomised trials." *The lancet* 378.9793 (2011): 771-784.

9. Holmes, Michelle D., et al. "Physical activity and survival after breast cancer diagnosis." *Jama* 293.20 (2005): 2479-2486.

10. King, A., MA, and Selak, and E. Gottlieb. "Succinate dehydrogenase and fumarate hydratase: linking mitochondrial dysfunction and cancer." *Oncogene* 25.34 (2006): 4675-4682.

11. Modica-Napolitano, Josephine S., and Keshav K. Singh. "Mitochondrial dysfunction in cancer." *Mitochondrion* 4.5 (2004): 755-762.

12. SINGH, KESHAV K. "Mitochondrial dysfunction is a common phenotype in aging and cancer." *Annals of the New York Academy of Sciences* 1019.1 (2004): 260-264.

13. Lin, Michael T., and M. Flint Beal. "Mitochondrial dysfunction and oxidative stress in neurodegenerative diseases." *Nature* 443.7113 (2006): 787-795.

14. Rucker, Robert, Winyoo Chowanadisai, and Masahiko Nakano. "Potential physiological importance of pyrroloquinoline quinone." *Alternative Medicine Review* 14.3 (2009): 268.

15. Chowanadisai, Winyoo, et al. "Pyrroloquinoline quinone stimulates mitochondrial biogenesis through cAMP response element-binding protein phosphorylation and increased PGC-1α expression." *Journal of Biological Chemistry* 285.1 (2010): 142-152.

16. Shults, Clifford W., et al. "Coenzyme Q10 levels correlate with the activities of complexes I and II/III in mitochondria from parkinsonian and nonparkinsonian subjects." *Annals of neurology* 42.2 (1997): 261-264.

17. Beal, M. Flint. "Mitochondrial dysfunction and oxidative damage in Alzheimer's and Parkinson's diseases and coenzyme Q10 as a potential treatment." *Journal of bioenergetics and biomembranes* 36.4 (2004): 381-386.

18. Long, Jiangang, et al. "Mitochondrial decay in the brains of old rats: ameliorating effect of alpha-lipoic acid and acetyl-L-carnitine." *Neurochemical research* 34.4 (2009): 755-763.

19. Timmers, Silvie, et al. "Calorie restriction-like effects of 30 days of resveratrol supplementation on energy metabolism and metabolic profile in obese humans." *Cell metabolism* 14.5 (2011): 612-622.

20. Pajuelo, David, et al. "Improvement of mitochondrial function in muscle of genetically obese rats after chronic supplementation with proanthocyanidins." *Journal of agricultural and food chemistry* 59.15 (2011): 8491-8498.

Endnote

This book summarizes some of the most effective natural therapies in the context of integrative oncology. Integrative oncology is a rapidly evolving field and I expect that future versions of this book will change as our understanding of integrative oncology advances. I am always striving to keep up with the research, and I am dedicated to understanding how natural medicines can be effectively integrated into a comprehensive treatment plan. The key to success is customizing a treatment plan that resonates most effectively with you, the patient. There are countless therapies that have positive studies supporting their use in cancer care. The challenge is sifting through this information to develop a targeted and simple plan for you.

Although the physical aspects of care are important, do not underestimate the power of the mind and the importance of emotions in your healing process. All of these critical components must be adequately addressed, and a Naturopathic doctor can help you develop an effective treatment plan. A Naturopathic doctor can act as an advocate for your health and ensure that you are getting the care that you need. These integrated plans are ultimately more effective than any single therapy on its own. When fighting any serious illness, do not base your hope on statistics. Hope is the variable that changes these statistics.

A

B

M

N

O

T

V

For the latest news and updates on
Integrative Oncology
visit the clinic website:

www.yaletownnaturopathic.com